Dancing With The Red Devil

Praise for Dancing With The Red Devil:

'A beautifully written gem of a book, both inspiring and poignant.' – *Elton John*

'Incisive and heart-rending.' – *Richard E. Grant*

'Sarah writes as she speaks: with down to earth honesty and self-deprecating wit. Not a whiff of burning martyr, and, if you ask me, *Dancing With The Red Devil* should be required reading for anyone whose life has been touched by cancer, and these days that's a hell of a lot of us!' – *Trisha Goddard*

'A tremendous book, and a remarkable testament to one woman's pluck, sense-of-humour and steely resolve.' – *William Boyd*

'Utterly wonderful. With comedy and candour Sarah has delivered a book that I will return to over and over again.' – *Susannah Constantine*

'A gloriously, infectiously irreverent manifesto in how to triumph against illness, this is writing of arresting fluency, brimming with laughter, of exquisite tenderness, courage and of the overwhelming impulse to grab life and LIVE. It's about the transcendent power of love, love of parent, spouse, child, grandchild, sibling, friend, and, above all, of life itself in all its disruptive and exhilarating complexity.' – *Juliet Nicolson*

'This is a book that makes you want to live and love every day.' – *Julia Samuel*

Dancing With The Red Devil

A Memoir of Love, Hope, Family and Cancer

SARAH STANDING

HEADLINE

First published in 2023 by
HEADLINE PUBLISHING GROUP

1

Cataloguing in Publication Data is available from the British Library

Hardback ISBN: 978 1 4722 9635 1

Typeset in 11/15pt Berling LT Std by Jouve (UK), Milton Keynes

Printed and bound in Great Britain by Clays Ltd, Elcograf S.p.A.

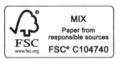

Headline's policy is to use papers that are natural, renewable and recyclable
products and made from wood grown in well-managed forests and other
controlled sources. The logging and manufacturing processes are expected
to conform to the environmental regulations of the country of origin.

HEADLINE PUBLISHING GROUP
An Hachette UK Company
Carmelite House
50 Victoria Embankment
London EC4Y 0DZ

www.headline.co.uk
www.hachette.co.uk

For my darling Dad. He always believed that I'd write a book one day, and I'm just sorry I didn't do it in his lifetime. This one is for you.

So we beat on, boats against the current, borne back ceaselessly into the past.

F. Scott Fitzgerald, *The Great Gatsby*

1

So imagine a Richard Curtis movie. Everybody can. They are a part of our DNA. There's the memorable, perfect music. The script that's pithy and current – it's not complicated or clever; watching each scene play out is just like overhearing a distant conversation that you can immediately identify with. People fuck up in Richard Curtis movies, but the right thing always happens in the end. This is my Richard Curtis movie. It's *my* movie, but I'm not sure I'm going to like the way it plays out. It's dark. It's like Quentin Tarantino queue-barged and muscled in without being invited. The fiction became pulped.

My film starts in London on an unnaturally crisp November day in 2020. The opening scene is promising. I get up, get dressed, go out and get an extra-hot, extra-shot flat white and go to work. I co-own a toy shop. A utopia of happiness. A place that gives me an enormous amount of pride and job satisfaction. It's a quirky, unique shop and working there is like living in a Technicolor fantasy world full of hope and dreams. I'm lucky – I look forward to going there every single day because, apart from anything else, I get to hang out with my best friend and co-owner, Diana, for five days a week.

We've known each other since our sons started school; and if you searched the globe for two women who were less alike, you'd end up casting us. I'm impetuous and loud and not great on detail. I overshare, show off and overembellish. Diana is methodical, constant and much more private than I. She's quality. She's kind. She's funny. She worries about things that don't even register on my radar, whilst I blunder on, impervious to impending disasters. We are the yin and yang of shopkeepers and yet, somehow, the perfect partners.

Every morning – in between blowing up helium balloons to tie outside the shop, and sipping coffee – we debrief. We have half an hour of what we call 'therapy'. We call it therapy with a deep sense of irony, because one of our running jokes is that we mock this endless quest for 'me time'. We're both in our sixties and 'me time' passed us by. As did extreme wokeness. And wearing gym clothes. And exercising at fancy gyms. We just walk. Fast.

We're the wrong generation, the wrong personalities, and had the wrong upbringing to comprehend – let alone embrace – any form of self-care or self-indulgence. We get a grip, suck it up, keep calm and carry on. Not because we're exceptional people, just because we've got no time. Running a shop, running a house, cooking, cleaning, shopping for food, taking care of husbands, grandchildren, dogs, dealing with grown-up children with grown-up problems; we're too busy being high-functioning enablers. We juggle. We often joke that by the time we get to work at nine in the morning, we've already showered, been to Waitrose, done two loads of laundry, made a fish pie, emptied the garbage, dealt with emails and walked the dog. Coming to work is our respite. It takes us away from domesticity and the middle-aged niggle of no longer having a full nest.

Diana and I run through the minutiae of our families with all the ease and speed of a child practising their piano scales before going to school. Gripes, gossip, dramas with children, dogs, what we cooked for dinner, who is annoying us, what we are doing at the weekend – it all tumbles out. We spend more time together than we do with our husbands, and consequently we have developed a fabulous, unjudgemental shorthand. After sixteen years of doing this together, Starbags is more than just a shop: it's our surrogate love child. Our sanity. Our escape.

Every day is showtime. The curtain goes up and the performance begins.

I'd been feeling breathless for about five days, and occasionally I was aware that my heart was maybe beating a bit too fast. Sometimes very fast. Scarily fast. It wasn't a pleasant feeling. At first, I put it down to a lack of sleep, or perhaps too much coffee. I tried to get an appointment with my NHS doctor but they weren't seeing patients in person, so they scheduled me in for a Zoom call. In six days' time. I am someone who is normally cavalier about my health, but this unnerved me. Five days . . . plus. Nearly a week. Too long.

I'm all about instant gratification. Hopeless at waiting. If I receive birthday presents in the post emblazoned with the plea 'NO PEEKING UNTIL YOUR BIRTHDAY', I open them immediately. I wake up in the mornings having slept for about four hours – five, if I'm on a lucky streak – and never pause, linger or snooze. I jump out of bed and am happily drinking my first cup of coffee within five minutes. If I ever get a cold – which I seldom do – I suffocate it with both Night and Day Nurse. And Nurofen Cold & Flu. I epitomise the impatient patient.

I went to a private GP, Christopher, whom I have seen, very occasionally, for years. He thought it was probably a nasty virus. He gave me antibiotics. And when those made no difference, he gave me a Covid test. Just to be safe. I forgot to say the backdrop to this movie is coronavirus. Fuck-struck coronavirus. Lord Covid is like a terrifying character from Harry Potter. One that wears an invisible cloak yet is omnipresent. My test came back negative. More antibiotics. But I was still breathless. He made me an appointment with a specialist, and by admitting he was at a loss as to what was causing my breathlessness, probably saved my life.

We've got through the first lockdown, lock-up, the interminable loss of freedom and friends, and the terrifying dystopian living nightmare that defined 2020. Now, despite being about to enter another circuit-breaking experiment (not quite as draconian as the first), Christmas is a-coming. Our shop is full of fake snow and fairy lights and although the government has decreed we must close in four days' time, we've defiantly declared that toy shops might not be considered essential, but Father Christmas is. He is without doubt a keyworker. We've promised all our customers that we will sell online, give virtual tours of the shelves, do click-and-collect sales from behind closed doors, and Instagram the hell out of our stock. Stockings will be filled. Not even Covid is going to get away with diluting children's dreams. Not on our watch.

So, I grab my glasses, my credit card and mask, hop into an Uber and speed off to meet a Dr Brian O'Conner at the Cromwell Hospital. A respiratory specialist. So certain am I that this is going to be a fast, expensive half-hour consultation, I don't even bother to take a handbag with me, I just shove everything into my coat pocket. It is a stunning November day. Blue skies.

The sort of day that makes one glad to be alive.

I check into reception, where I am heat-scanned before being handed a pristine paper mask by a woman holding a yard-long pair of tweezers. Contactless. At this point during the pandemic, everything in the hospital is distanced. The floor resembles a giant game of Twister with huge, circular discs. There are red circles to stand on whilst you wait to get your sticker saying 'Screening

Completed', before you are ushered off to stand on a blue circle. Then you shuffle on to yellow, while your registration is processed.

I have an overwhelming desire to try to reach the next level before it's my turn. To cheat. To do the splits, keeping one foot on blue whilst sliding my leg over to the yellow. It now takes longer to get into a hospital department than it did to gain entry to my favourite club, Studio 54 in New York, back in the day. You have to pass selection. But the nightclub clipboard Nazis (as they were known) have been replaced by hospital prefects officiously moving the patients along. Before long, I'm in the system. Shuffling along, sticking to the rules, not overstepping the mark, getting my credit card details logged, being asked if I'm displaying any Covid symptoms. Moving along the Covid conveyor belt. I get the obligatory sticker saying 'Screening Completed', which reminds me of going to the dentist as a small child. The reward for being good and compliant – a badge of honour.

Dr O'Conner is a Norman Rockwell kind of guy. Old school. A proper doc. Calm. Methodical. My age. Polite. Reassuring. I tell him I take no medication. No statins. No HRT. No nothing. I've had antibiotics about eight times in my life. I care about my health, but it's yet to interrupt me and test my mortality.

He examines me. Starts the slow hands-on-the-body routine.

'Does this feel swollen to you?' he asks, pressing under my ribs.

'Not really.'

'How about here?' he asks, moving slightly downwards. 'Notice a feeling of slight fullness?'

'A bit,' I say, having a sudden flashback to the numerous nights I've made myself a hot-water bottle at 3 a.m. and gone back to sleep, hugging it for comfort, because perhaps I did have a slight feeling of . . . what was it? Fullness. That's what it felt like. It *was* fullness.

'Okay,' says Dr O'Conner, springing back to his desk. He starts scribbling. 'You are going to go back to the main hospital and I'm going to arrange for an ultrasound, an X-ray and extensive blood tests, and then I want you to come back to me, and I can look at the results.'

Back I go. I genuinely feel no sense of foreboding. I'm such an innocent when it comes to medical tests. I've never really needed any of consequence. I just assume Dr O'Conner is being professional and cautious before sending me away with a prescription for strong antibiotics and a hefty invoice. So I merrily go back to playing Twister. Red circle, yellow circle. Pause. X-ray. Bloods. Ultrasound. The last time I was in hospital for anything was thirty-one years ago today. No joke. On 3 November 1989, I gave birth to Tilly, my youngest child. Epidural. No pain, just gain.

The ultrasoundist (is that even a word?) glides his probe over my stomach and then stops. Prods deeper. Slithers over my flab and then stops again. The screen is facing away from me.

'Who's your oncologist?' he asks nonchalantly.

I wipe off the jelly that is dripping down my stomach. 'My oncologist?' I ask. 'Oh, I don't have an oncologist. I don't have anything that wrong with me. No, I'm just here seeing Dr O'Conner to sort out my breathlessness.'

No alarm bells ring. Not one. Not even a muffled tinkle.

I'm just here for the quick fix. Nothing more. A second opinion and then home. And anyway, Richard Curtis would never, ever have given away the plot this early on in any one of his films. Much too corny. As improbable as it seems, given the beauty of hindsight, I just completely disregard the comment. It totally passes me by. This guy is obviously reading from the wrong script. Not one meant for me.

Back to Dr O'Conner's office.

He's waiting for me. Standing up. He's got images of me up on his screen. He's leaning over his laptop. Studying. Studying my innards. Blurry black and white shapes. Light and dark.

'Well, well. I wasn't expecting this,' he says. 'No wonder you've been feeling breathless. There's a lot of fluid in here. See this?' He points to the screen. 'It's pressing against your lungs. It's pushing up on all your organs. We need to drain that off.'

'How do you do that?' I ask, with all the innocence of a woman who's made it to sixty-one without a broken bone or a single stitch to her body.

'Very simple procedure; we just put a thin wire in and aspirate the liquid,' he replies. 'I've arranged for it to be done immediately – they are waiting for you in the main hospital.'

Aspirate. All these medical terms are new to me.

Simple procedures are all relative, but I now know that, medically speaking, a 'simple procedure' is a mere euphemism for something fucking painful that is done with only a local anaesthetic. Everyone inflicting this pain acts as though what is about to happen is as ordinary, and as uneventful, as having your nails painted.

First, I slip out of my clothes and into a hospital gown. I get on to a trolley and nurses ask me questions and I sign a consent form. Contact numbers. Next of kin. Known allergies. A shiny, printed identification band is attached to my wrist with my name, date of birth and hospital number.

The doctor comes in. Starts copping a feel of bits of my body. Squeezing flesh. Looking for easy entry points. I force myself to try to disengage from whatever it is that is about to happen to me. I look up at the ceiling. I silently hum. Pretending my mind is separated from my body. Now I'm cuffed and my blood pressure is being taken, my pulse monitored. My body is manually shifted until it's in a good position to gain an entry point.

The onslaught begins.

'Just a little sting,' says the doctor, injecting me with a local anaesthetic. 'And another little prick coming up now.'

Now my mask is slipping. I'm sweating. I realise the two nurses are the politically correct version of human straitjackets. In the olden days they'd have restrained me for this 'procedure', for the safety of both the doctor and themselves. Because if I weren't polite, and if I weren't relatively well brought up, I'd have kicked him in the balls by now and rendered him permanently infertile. Instead, I pant and make tiny talk.

I talk about the Trump–Biden election, which is taking place tonight, as though I have a deeply vested interest in the outcome. Displacement tactics. I apologise for being a bit of a wimp. Turns out the two stings were just the precursor before the main event. Jesus. Silly me. The wire has to go in and be threaded God knows where inside my body, in order to aspirate whatever it is that needs to be aspirated.

'I'm so sorry, I'm so sorry,' I say, big fat tears rolling into my face mask.

What am I actually sorry for? I'm so sorry for feeling pain. So sorry that I'm not braver and that I'm white-knuckling it. I'm so sorry I'm jerking when the needle goes in, and for not staying statue-still. I'm so sorry I'm crying.

'You're doing really well,' says the nurse, whilst methodically stroking my clawed hand.

But I'm not. Truth be told, I'm not doing well at all. They're just flattering me. Everything is taking place behind my back, so I have no idea how close to ending this 'little procedure' is. And I'm suddenly scared. I'm out of my safety zone. I really have no clue what is happening to me. And I wish, more than anything, there was someone who loved me in the waiting room, ready to give me a reassuring hug when it's all over.

'Nearly done,' says the doctor, before another agonising five minutes of foraging about. 'Now, I just need to stick this down and make sure it's secure. There. All done.'

I sit up and thank him profusely. So English.

I now have a bag of what looks exactly like Daylesford's organic bone broth attached to me. It's dripping out of my body. Plop. Plop. Plop. Slowly filling up a transparent bag nestled in the bed beside me.

I can't help but think of the irony. Thirty-one years ago today, I had my new baby, Tilly – my last baby – snuggled beside me. Tilly with her perfect rosebud mouth and fierce, dark quiff of hair. Swaddled, immobile and unable to flail. A little parcel of perfection I could prop up on my knees to study every feature of her adorable face, smell her specialness and imprint both on to my soul. But no baby this time.

Today, I just have bone broth.

The good news – and God knows one always has to remember to search for the good news – is I can now breathe easy. I'm not breathless any more. Suddenly, I'm aware that I've been holding my breath for the last three weeks.

Making my bed required too much effort. Walking in the park every other morning with my great friend Anya was too hard. One day, holding my delicious nine-month-old grandson Billy required Herculean strength.

My son Archie dropped Billy at my shop for half an hour – for me to take care of him whilst he went to have his tyre fixed. As soon as he left, I realised I had to make Billy safe. I had to wedge him into a cardboard box with a cushion, because carrying him made my heart pump out of control. I was really scared I would drop him. Running downstairs to the stockroom in the shop required acting. On the way back up, I lingered on the top step, trying to catch my breath in an abortive attempt to regain my composure. Acting. I was putting on a performance. Pretending all was okay. Fooling myself.

Me and my bone broth go off to have another scan. Arms up, bracelets off, necklace taped out of the way. The dull hum of machinery rumbling above my head.

Teatime and by now I'm checked in to the hospital.

I'm a patient. I lie on the bed fully clothed. I stare at the watercolour opposite my bed. I drink bottle after bottle of water because my mouth is dry with fear and adrenaline, and I watch *Sky News*. My eldest, ever-practical daughter, India, drops off a phone charger at reception. She can't come up to see me. Covid rules. The phone charger is a game changer. Every so often a nurse comes in and drains the broth out, and then I watch, mesmerised, as the bag slowly refills. What is this foreign liquid?

It's getting dark. The gloaming. No idea when I'm going home. All the broth has to drain out of my body first. That's the deal.

Sky News drones on and I fiddle about with my phone.

Dr O'Conner comes in. Delicately takes my big-girl knickers and my trousers off the chair where I've flung them, and sits down. He's got two masks on and a plastic visor and a rubber apron and gloves.

'Mind if I switch the television off?' he asks.

'Be my guest.'

'I hate all this mask business,' he says apologetically. 'I hate having to keep my distance. Um, I'm not that sort of doctor.'

I nod in agreement. Spit it out, I think. Cut to the chase. I want to continue watching the election.

He pauses and looks me directly in the eye. Hands folded.

'You've got cancer. It's the best possible cancer you could have at your age, but it's quite large and I think it's pressing against your kidneys.'

I've gone back to being a little bit breathless. I don't say anything. I just look up at the curtain softly flapping, and I flick my foot against the sheet. I feel like my soul and heart are on the ceiling, only my body is left lying passively on the bed. I am floating about. I am the Debra Winger character in the 1993 movie *Shadowlands* (about C. S. Lewis's relationship with the much younger American writer Joy Davidman) and Dr O'Conner is Anthony Hopkins, but without the hand-holding. They were lovers in the movie. She died.

'Further tests will show if it's Hodgkin's or non-Hodgkin's lymphoma, and . . .'

But I've vagued off. I don't hear any more medical

words. I keep having strange thoughts. Displaced thoughts. Hodgkin's or non-Hodgkin's. To be or not to be. Hodgkin's or non-Hodgkin's. I think of music. A soundtrack to my very own personal movie. Adele is right here in the room next to me, swaying and swishing her skirt. It's loud. Together, we are 'Rolling in the Deep'.

'I'm worried about your husband,' continues Dr O'Conner, looking at me intently, trying to gauge my state of mind. 'I think this is going to be very hard on him.'

He knows Johnnie. My rock. The love of my life for nearly forty years. He made Johnnie better last year, when he had a chest infection. He gave him steroids and cured him.

'I know,' I say. 'I am worried too. Because I'm twenty-five years younger than he. And I guess if you marry someone twenty-five years younger than you, this isn't really part of the game plan. I've fucked up. I was supposed to be the one who took care of him, not the other way around.'

There is a long, pregnant pause. I don't cry.

I can hear the trolley with dinner on it trundling down the passage. A buzzer goes off at the end of the corridor. The curtain flaps. The room gets darker.

'No,' agrees Dr O'Conner. 'I understand what you are saying. But this is a good cancer to have at your age and . . .'

And . . . and . . . and up to the ceiling I go again.

And I'm sure we talk some more, and I assume I ask questions, and I'm sure I am given some instructions and information. And I know he is being kind. I will never forget how kind he is. He is really, really kind.

But I blank it. All of it. I blank it.

Because I know I have to somehow find a steely calm and resolve. My fear will have to be put on pause, because I know that as soon as he leaves me alone, I have to pick up the phone and, one by one, make every single member of my family unbelievably sad.

I have to break their once happy hearts with an ice pick.

2

I go into the bathroom. I need to first rehearse my lines before I tackle telling my family. I look at myself in the mirror. I lean in and look into my eyes. But my eyes have died. My pupils are big, blank and dull. I don't recognise the person I'm looking at. I desperately need a script to follow. I have no idea how to play this. I can't just ad-lib; I need a plan. I give myself options. Lines I could use.

'Hi. Don't quite know how to put this, but I have cancer.' No. Too brutal.

'Hey, guys. Listen, the doctor has just been – and guess what? I've gone and done something really stupid. I've got cancer.' Too flip.

'Fuck. You will never guess what? Do you want to hear the good news or the bad news first?' Too obvious. Too corny. Even Hugh Grant would baulk at that one.

And does the fact I supposedly have a 'good' cancer really qualify for good news? What the hell is a 'good'

SARAH STANDING

cancer anyway? I thought they were all, by definition, fuckers.

In the end, I decide on simply, 'I'm sorry.' I am sorry.

I'm sorry for myself, and I'm sorry I've ruined everything. And I'm really sorry I'm probably going to lose all my hair before Christmas. And I'm sorry I've got an eighty-six-year-old husband whom I adore and who can't cook anything except toast and eggs, and doesn't know how to work the washing machine. He needs me to be healthy and strong – as does my eighty-six-year-old mother, who lives alone and who doesn't know how to use a mobile phone or buy what she wants on Amazon. I promised my dad I would always be there for her, take care of her. They need me. They both need me.

And I have three grown-up children who probably *don't* need me any more, yet I love them so much it hurts. And I'm so sorry that I'm going to have to reverse roles and need them. I don't want them to be burdened with me. I'm sorry I'm going to morph into the bore they must check up on and run errands for. And sorry I'm going to be the granny who's temporarily too bald and too tired to babysit.

I'm sorry I won't be able to work with Diana in our shop, if lockdown ever ends. Nor will I have the energy to walk with Anya on cold, misty mornings, storming around Battersea Park. And I'm furious with my sister Emma for living in America because I know if it weren't for fuck-struck Covid she'd immediately get on the next plane out and fly over, with loads of the cheap Sea Breeze astringent from CVS drugstore I've used since I was a teenager to

17

take off my make-up. It appals her, she considers it just below paint stripper. But I know she'd bring it. And cosy pyjamas, crap magazines and Life Savers sweets. Above all, she would make me laugh. And just be with me.

She'd give our mum a false, positive spin on my diagnosis. One she could live with. Keep her calm. Our mum, Nanette Newman, doesn't really accept death as an inevitability, as a natural consequence of living. She considers it optional. She never accepted the fact that our dad was dying. She would greet doctors by saying, 'I only want to hear the good news,' so they were left telling her only what she wanted to hear. Emma and I had to keep the bad news to ourselves. And that was a heavy burden to carry. The pretence.

I need my sister to be my wingman. To hold my hand. To hear the bad news. To share the load. But she can't. She's trapped in another lockdown. In another country. Another spunk-hole of star-spangled Hades across the seas. If I ask her to come to me, she will have to turn her back on her family. Her kids. Her husband. I can't ask that of her. And anyway, Covid has virtually all but blackballed international travel.

I walk slowly back from the bathroom, and sit on the edge of my bed. Elton and Bernie got it right. Sorry does seem to be the hardest word.

I call Johnnie.

'Sorry, but I've gone and done something really, really cuntish,' I say quickly. I spit it out. 'I've got cancer.'

There. I've done it. I've said it. I've destroyed him. One small sentence. Worse than any spiteful row at 2 a.m., worse than the time I hit him in a fury, worse than the time I threatened to walk out and never come back. I've not just destroyed him; I've triple-dared him. I've made him promise to tell our three children for me. I'm brave, but alas, I'm not that brave.

Our children are our life. India, Archie and Tilly. All uniquely different; each of them savagely dissimilar, in both personality and temperament.

India, our eldest, is independent, stylish, un-needy, pragmatic, practical, loyal and irreverent. She never really embraced childish things – including, and especially, school. Given a choice, she liked to wear black as a little girl. An individual from an early age who never got involved with peer pressure. Precociously verbal, as opposed to physical, she barely bothered to walk until she was nearly two, and was totally disinterested in crawling. She was at her happiest talking and would fight against being part of a clan. She's always been safe in her own skin. Secure.

She called us twelve years ago to tell us she was getting married. In America. In two days' time. Only wanted the groom to be there. Didn't ever want a big event; never wanted all eyes to be on her. Being the centre of attention didn't appeal. Never dreamt about a big puffy dress and wedding bells. She's private. Contained. It temporarily broke my heart, as I so wanted to witness the partial parental full stop that comes with an offspring's wedding ceremony; yet equally I had to respect her reasoning. She'd applied a typically unsentimental and practical approach. She was marrying a divine American photographer called Sean Thomas; having navigated a transatlantic relationship for two years, they both needed the freedom and security of being able to spend long periods of time together, without fighting the authorities for visas.

She knew her mum and dad were going through a financial fallow patch, and was mindful of our circumstances. They both adhered to the reasoning of 'all for one and one for all'. If they invited us, they would have to invite Sean's parents, and all their siblings and their partners, and, and, and . . . And then it would become a proper, traditional shindig. Neither of them was up for that. So instead, they got married at an office in Long Island, with zero pomp and ceremony. Low key. India's best friend was already there, as was Sean's, and they acted as witnesses. A bouquet of white hydrangeas, a wedding snap taken on their way back into New York, alongside a massive, life-size T-rex, in bed by 9 p.m. with a bottle of champagne and a takeaway. Like Frank, she did it her way.

Six months later, we threw them a party at our house. And the original full stop that had clogged my heart faded forever into a mere comma. One of those familial stories that make up the patchwork quilt of life. They are parents to our first glorious grandson, Huck.

Archie, our middle child, born thirteen months after India, was always fanatical about sport. As a baby he used to take a ball to bed with him; never a teddy. When

I reminisce and look back at his childhood, it was always about sport. He used to cry when Chelsea lost; and to this day, it's wise not to talk to him for a good two hours after an unsuccessful game. But cricket was his true love, his passion. He was exceptionally gifted at it, but he also opened his arms wide to embrace rugby, football, golf, tennis – and shone effortlessly at all of them. I had no brothers (yet always longed for one) and was utterly besotted by his innate maleness, although wilfully ill-equipped, too inexperienced and too girly to be a good touchline mother. I'm sure I was an embarrassment at times. Overly cautious. I used to stand in my thoroughly inappropriate stilettoes (which would sink into the sodden pitch), watching him play rugby and shouting embarrassing instructions like 'Drop the ball!' because I was always terrified he'd be tackled and get hurt. Arch, to be fair, never held this against me. Possibly because I was also unaware it was against the rules to hand out cigarettes to his fellow seventeen-year-old pupils whilst sunbathing on the roof of the cricket pavilion, hanging out with the boys waiting to go into bat. Archie wears his heart on his sleeve. He's articulate, emotional, kind and ridiculously responsible. A rock of a man – and now, with his partner Nisha, a sensational father to Billy.

Born just three days before the first lockdown, both of them had to navigate the first weeks of hazy parenthood with no help whatsoever. It broke my heart. I first hugged Billy in Chelsea and Westminster with a mask on and then was prevented from snuggling him properly for weeks. FaceTime only. Nisha and Archie coped with no help in a foreign, scary, uncertain, fucked-up landscape. Nisha was a total Trojan. The most selfless mother a child could wish for. It is my deepest regret I couldn't be more hands on. I was totally useless. Redundant. They both went through the baptism of fire that is parenthood alone. I take my hat off to them. Not easy. Archie is a confident parent, and Nisha is a calm and patient one. Great combo. Billy is a lucky boy.

And then there's Tilly, our youngest. Her first sentence was a question, and indicative of her innate sweetness. 'Are you 'appy?' She's sentimental and thoughtful, with massive emotional intelligence. Full of self-deprecating funniness. She was a very lush baby. Full lipped, and the dark quiff of hair she was born with faded into a little halo of blond curls. She was also a perfectionist who would make me endlessly redo her ponytail before school, and a kid who would get frustrated when covering her textbooks with sticky-backed plastic if there was a single pop of an air bubble. Tilly has an effortless ability to not only be a great friend, but also to have an army of friends who adore her back. She thinks deeply about things. When she was five, she asked me if I would rather she were crucified or died a natural death.

And now, I am about to ruin her birthday by crucifying her.

And Johnnie. Sadly, I can visualise him swallowing this news. Alone. In our home. With no one to hold him. He told me later – much, much later – that he lay on our bed and howled. And he also told me he hadn't cried for over fifty years. Stiff upper lip and all that. It broke my heart.

So thank you, Covid. You are the gift that just keeps on giving. I have to drop this C-bomb into a phone call, like a casual lunch invitation. I am allowed no visitors. No hugging. No human touch. Not today. Not tonight. Not tomorrow. Already, brimming with self-pity, I hate Covid more than I hate cancer.

Covid is making me go through this alone.

Now I am a callous assassin. I'm like an avatar on *Fortnite* – I'm a storm trooper, armed and picking off people with my bad news.

I text my brother-in-law, Graham, in Long Island and ask him to call me ASAP. Which he does. Graham must have read the urgency in my text, because he works harder than anyone I know. Covid and lockdown hasn't made him miss a beat; he just has uninterruptable Zoom meetings from dawn until dusk, with my sister sliding meals on to his desk out of sight of the camera.

He calls me immediately. Sweet, kind, ever pragmatic, Graham takes the news and reacts perfectly. I feed off his calm. We perform a perfect duet of strategic damage control. I don't want my sister to be alone when I tell her. I need him to catch her if she falls.

I call Anya. Call Diana. Call one of my oldest friends, Reidy.

No preamble. Like reading a bad bedtime story you know is going to give children hideous nightmares, I plough on. I don't edit out the nasty bits. I don't bother. I tell them like it is. I invite the bogeyman in. Reidy is lost for words. He can't take it in. He says he will call me later. Anya has to pull over from driving, to talk to me through tears. And Diana is Diana. Solid. Steadying.

The thing is, I love life. Everyone says that, but what I really mean is, I love *my* life. I love everything about it, starting at the top. I love my country. I love my house. I love my neighbourhood, my shops, my job, my parks, my routine. I love the tiny pot-planted wilderness I've nurtured outside my front door. I love the fact I have collected over twenty-five different-coloured pairs of Converse sneakers. I love the colour on our drawing-room walls: Grenville pink. I love the way the rain sometimes wakes me up by splatting on to my skylight windows above my bed. I love an awful lot. But most of all, I love the people in my life. My family. My friends. They are my oxygen.

And I am enveloped in love, back. It drowns me. Suffocates me. Down the telephone wires, I feel nothing but this tsunami of strength gathering force. I may be alone in a shitty A-line hospital gown, I may be lying on a bed with a rubber mattress beneath me, I may have bone broth flowing out of my side, and I may be watching Trump behaving like a spoilt loser on TV, with the volume turned right down, but I don't feel alone. I feel like I've amassed a loyal army by my side.

Fuck it. Fuck you, cancer. Fuck you, Covid. I genuinely don't have time for any of this. Nor do my family and friends, by the sound of it. We are not interested in cancer's intrusive takeover bid. It can try to take me hostage, but I absolutely refuse to give in to its demands.

I decide, there and then, that I will never allow it to define me. This is not who I am.

What I am, though, is a woman being asked for an anal swab. Another part of hospital procedure, waging a war on some kind of MRSA. So into the bathroom I go, with Vince, a fabulously attractive French nurse.

I need Adele to come with me for this one. She's 'Rolling in the Deep' beside me. The pounding, internal soundtrack to my newfound situation; momentarily distracting me from all that I have suddenly become.

I could have had it all. Indeed, this morning, I did.

That first night, I sit bolt upright in bed with the American election on mute. I don't sleep. I'm plotting the middle bit of my Richard Curtis movie. It's taken a bit of a dark turn. I start writing. I feel an overwhelming desire to get my emotions down, in order to somehow make some sense of what is happening to me. It's an old trick I learnt long ago. Get my raw feelings out of my head and on to paper. I write in order to find out what I'm thinking, without the agony of saying it out loud. Diluting the thoughts helps. A bit. Written words are somehow less violent.

After less than twenty-four hours in hospital, I'm already fully institutionalised. My body is just a vessel. It's not the same body that danced to Abba at my sixtieth birthday party in sparkly Lurex trousers and high-heeled platform shoes. It's not the body that watched television documentaries whilst giving birth, because I chose to have epidurals pretty much as soon as I entered the car park. It's not the body that's got little wrists and dry skin between my toes. It's not the same body my husband used to say had the softest skin he'd ever felt. Nor is it the same body that always just did as it was told. It's morphed. It's a medical mess. It belongs to someone else. Not me.

Post-breakfast, I'm disconnected from the tube coming out of my back. I'm slightly disconcerted that the two nurses who arrive to get it out have to google the right way to do the procedure on their iPhones. They are arguing behind my back about the width of the tube, because that determines the exit plan. And it hurts coming out, no lie.

I'm measured and weighed, and I'm pushed into lifts and taken off for scans and MRIs and to have blood taken and for another, much worse, 'simple procedure'. It's like being a contestant on *I'm a Celebrity . . . Get Me Out of Here!* – endless bushtucker trials and tests of stamina.

Today's task is a biopsy, done by a female doctor who says, 'Goodie, you are nice and thin, which makes my job so much easier.'

I've never cared about a compliment less.

I'm thrilled. Thrilled that after two little 'stings' – one to numb my flank, followed by another 'slightly deeper' little sting – she thinks she'll be able to get easy access to take slivers of my tumour.

Two nurses come in. I call them 'the Placaters'. One

strokes my forehead with blue rubber-gloved hands, whilst the other monitors my blood pressure.

Then the doctor starts. This is the worst 'procedure' yet. And it takes an inordinate amount of time. Too much time.

'How much longer?' I ask, frantically trying to keep my shit together. 'How much longer? How many more minutes?' I'm shaking.

This old vessel is already starting to list.

Back in my room, I wait to meet my oncologist for the first time. He's late. He whizzes in with his hands full of files and his mobile in his hand. A Nokia. A no-frills Nokia. Old school. He's hesitant, slight, dishevelled and unassuming. A man on a mission.

He flicks through my notes with alacrity. It's like being with a headmaster going through my school report. Geography – fine. English – not bad. Maths – needs improvement. Flick, flick, flick. A pink note flutters to the floor.

Dr Plowman looks up. 'Ninety per cent certain what we're dealing with here is a non-Hodgkin's tumour, it's perching on your kidney. You will need chemo – probably six sessions. These sorts of large tumours react very quickly to treatment.'

'Where would I be treated?'

'Here. At the Cromwell.'

'Will I resent you for having just spent a fortune having my highlights done?'

'Yes. But your hair will grow back.'

'How fast will I lose it?'

'After about two sessions.'

My own GP warned me that I might not warm to Plowman's bedside manner. He said he's a very matter-of-fact doctor. But I actually like matter-of-fact. I've found I don't respond to fluffy good-news bandits. Nor do I respond to wrapping up bad news. I'm a journalist. I deal in hard facts. I've had a career littered with rejections and un-returned phone calls. I react best to certainties.

'He's direct,' said Christopher.

I like direct. I like the fact that every nurse, when asked who my oncologist is, has sort of quivered with deep respect. 'Dr Plowman is fabulous,' they say, as though letting me into a deep secret. 'You are lucky.'

Up until this point in my life, my definition of luck has followed a slightly different trajectory. I was always lucky with cards. Blackjack. I was lucky with the weather when I went on holiday. I once was supremely lucky picking the Grand National winner, despite the fact I had zero knowledge of racing whatsoever. I was lucky when it came to love. I was lucky in that I managed to write for every publication I ever aspired to write for. The *Telegraph*, the *Spectator*, *Condé Nast Traveller*, *The Times*. I was lucky in that I had a happy childhood, with parents who loved each other. That I was still married and had succeeded in giving my children stability and security. I had a lovely life. I was spoilt with luck.

And now, I am going to be lucky in that I'm getting an oncologist who will pump me full of chemotherapy and indirectly make me lose my hair. A different type of luck.

'I need to tell you something about myself, Dr Plowman,' I say, getting off the bed to deliver the speech I want to give, my bare arse exposed. This wasn't rehearsed. 'I've been married for nearly forty years to a man I love, we have three children, two grandchildren, and I love my life. I've been a journalist for thirty years and I co-own a toyshop. I've decided I am never, ever going to google anything about this disease, nor am I ever going to listen to anyone who tries to tell me they have a second cousin once removed with the same cancer. I think doing either of those things could take me to a dark place. I also imagine cancer is much the same as fingerprints. Everyone's completely unique.'

He looks up from his notes. 'In that case,' he says, 'you sound like my perfect patient. You do your job and I'll do mine. I know what I'm doing.'

I can tell he's smiling through his mask. We bump elbows.

Fuck Covid. Fuck cancer.

I trust him. I must. I have no other choice: I have to trust him with my life.

3

Back home, I wait for more news, hovering between the life I knew before and an unknown world I'm about to enter. None of it seems real. It reminds me of when I was once in a minor earthquake in Los Angeles. Before it happened, everything was normal. And then the earth moved, but not in an orgasmic way. It wasn't overly dramatic. It was a bit like smoking grass, back in the day, when drugs were pure, homegrown, fun and a laugh. Slow-motion reactions at first. Quite pleasant. Then . . . *boom!* The floor suddenly turned to jelly. For thirty seconds everything went wobbly and felt ominously psychedelic. Getting a cancer diagnosis feels like that. I have crossed the Rubicon. I feel destabilised. Very discombobulated. Floating. Present but not present. Like I'm in a holding pattern. I'm circling; just like aeroplanes do, dumping excess fuel in order to land. It makes me feel a little bit queasy.

Parts of my life remain totally normal. I'm attempting to micro-manage the shop from home. I'm basting salmon with ginger and soy sauce, I'm bunging a baked potato in the oven for supper, I'm putting the rubbish out. I'm doing a jigsaw at night with Johnnie and watching *The Chase*. I'm playing Woodoku on my iPhone and I'm plucking stray hairs from my chin. I'm doing mundane stuff. And I'm going to bed with a sleeping pill and failing miserably to sleep.

My days are jam packed. Appointments. Admin. Markers. Covid tests. Bloods. Every day, I get forms, bills. Phone calls from unknown numbers pop up and I can't just flip them off. They are all coming from doctors, secretaries, people who want my date of birth and my credit card details.

My medical insurance company has informed me they don't cover cancer. Cheers. I took out the policy when I was twenty-five and was a young, near-perfect specimen. I never read the small print, nor made a single claim, until I was nearly forty and had a weird, potentially cancerous mole that turned out to be benign. Back then, I felt invincible. And now that I am flawed and broken and in need, they are turning their back on me. Were I to be involved in a major accident, require a new hip, or suddenly need to have a colonoscopy, they would stand and deliver. But not now. Long-term cancer treatment involving chemo, no can do. They don't want to know. They will pick up the tab for one scan, but that's going to be a piss in the ocean.

Time is of the essence. I recognise that if I go the NHS route, I might end up dead. There is a sense of overwhelming urgency attached to receiving a cancer diagnosis. No hanging about. Deal with it. Now. No lingering.

My dad left me some money in his will, with the codicil it was 'for a rainy day' – and I reckon this is my monsoon. I justify my profligate attitude and privilege by coming to terms with the fact I am freeing up a bed for someone else who doesn't have a dad who left them a small legacy. Once I've come to that decision and made peace with it, and accepted the fact there is no turning back, I reach a point of acceptance. Life is teetering on the cusp of being short. My life. I want, I need, mine to be longer. Sixty-one years isn't long enough.

I view myself as just brushing mid-life, not duelling with end-of-life. I still wear blue jeans that are ripped, buy *Grazia* magazine religiously and like Cheesy Wotsits. I unattractively chew gum and am partial to lying to my children about how much SPF I use when sunbathing. I dream of buying a 1950s caravan, decking it out and taking it to Cornwall. Obviously, I *am* a grown-up, but I sure as shit don't feel like one.

Not yet. Not me.

Alongside the arse-paralysing admin, the weirdest thing happens. Overnight, I become the star of my own fan club. An epic fan club, gaining momentum every day. A bit like when Facebook was first launched: You joined, made a friend request to six people, and fired up your laptop the next morning to discover that, like sap rising, your network had magically expanded. Gone ballistic.

New members joined with the alacrity of fast-moving lava. It's the same with cancer. You tell a few people, and within twenty-four hours you are a cancer celebrity. Starring in, producing and directing your very own medical drama.

It seems everyone I've ever known wants to audition for a bit part. I've become an overnight sensation: a diva. A prima donna. Full of demands that I'm not making, but people are offering to fulfil. I'm lapping it up with disbelief, wonder and gratitude.

A couple of reactions take me by surprise. 'Your secret is safe with me; I promise I won't tell anyone.' Why? I don't have some embarrassing STD: I'm just the boring statistical one out of two people for whom the bell has tolled. I'm the one. My number came up. I have cancer. There is no secret to keep, I reassure them. I'm going for full disclosure. Tell whom you like.

Friends are so kind, so thoughtful, so articulate in coming forward and telling me how they feel about me. Offering to help. It's humbling. Truly humbling. Every text is like a soundbite from an obituary I would never in normal circumstances get to read. They make me cry. I receive flowers and food and parcels and messages and cards and emails and letters. I treasure them. It's so good to talk. With no hugs, no touching and no visitors, words are my only distraction. I have to be so careful that Johnnie (because of his age) is shielded from Covid, as well: neither of us can afford to take risks. Can't let people into our house, for fear they might be carriers, incubating the dreaded virus. Our bubble has popped and has just become a whole lot tinier. We are both living like hermits.

On the other hand, life itself has become less mundane with cancer thrown into the mix. Even bigger. More dramatic. More newsworthy. Lockdowns, shielding, Covid and social distancing make life not just scary, but dull. Monumentally dull. So boring. There's been so little to talk about. With anyone. Main topics of conversation have revolved around recipes, Netflix, gardening, wistful plans of moving to the country, Cummings, Boris, Trump, Hancock, vaccines, clapping, Captain Tom, Piers Morgan, and going to bed at 9 p.m. Most marriages have been reduced to a series of grunts whilst watching the telly and being disproportionately jealous when your spouse's mobile rings.

There is very little to say, without individual daily adventures: the work dramas, the walks, the bumping into people, the dinner parties, the gossip, the unexpected. Normal life may frequently have seemed like a daily grind, but compared to Covid confinement, it was the highlife. We were all living the dream. Going to work, looking forward to holidays, theatre outings, booking a manicure, going to a movie, a restaurant, a shop. Oh, how we took these things for granted.

We have spent the last ten months on pause. In suspended animation, with precious little movement. Waiting for the Amazon and Ocado delivery men to ring the bell. Waiting to mark off another Thursday by going outside with a saucepan and clapping for the NHS and shouting hello to a neighbour across the road. That's it. A little life. A very tiny, squeezed life.

Domestic conversations reduced to, 'Let me take the rubbish out, it will give me something to do.'

'No, I will. You did it last time.'

'Let's not argue. Let's do it together.'

God forbid one of us misses out on an 'activity' to break up the monotony.

Scrolling through the contacts on our phones, trying to find someone new to ring. Listening to each other's conversations; hungry, starving, lustful for fresh news. The oxygen of hope.

'Tell me all your news,' my mother has said, every day, when I ring up to check on her.

'I have none,' I've replied, truculently. It reminds me of being asked as a child what I did at school.

I envy those with continuing, time-consuming jobs who are busy Zooming, and conference-calling, and 'WFH', and bothering to put on mascara. Keeping up appearances. My shop is just closed. Shut. *Fermé*. With decorative Santas and penguins gathering dust amongst the fake snow and the fairy lights twinkling in the windows. I haven't done all the things I've always said I'd do if I had more time. I've had all the time in the world, yet I haven't learnt a new language, read the pile of books beside my bed, filled my photograph albums, taken up needlepoint. I haven't even made banana bread. Shame on me.

But now at least my cancer has given everyone something to talk about – most of all me. I do have news.

Breaking news. And I'm up for a chat. I'm up all night sometimes, as I'm still circling, and unable to sleep. I love the fact my sister is in America and is five hours behind me. I FaceTime her for hours, and I am therefore not alone. I have an umbilical cord of familial night-time love to keep me sane during the endless witching hours.

But. But. There is always a big but. There is still one more procedure I need to have before 'the Big Reveal', as my son has nicknamed next Tuesday night's meeting with Dr Plowman, my oncologist. The gathering of information, the definitive test results. The fingers-crossed, hoping-against-hope verdict that I'm harbouring a 'contained' cancer. I'm going to be allowed to bring both Johnnie and Archie to the Big Reveal. Masked and sanitised, obviously, but they have been given special dispensation to attend, so that they can make notes, ask questions, and witness me being handed down my sentence.

But first, I must have the mother of all bushtucker trials: the bone marrow biopsy/harvesting/lumbar puncture thing. The biggie. The 'procedure' that gives even my own seasoned GP the willies, when I ask him about it.

An incredibly nice Jordanian doctor does it. I went to Jordan once – another lifetime ago. I visited both Aqaba and Petra. It was the first time I'd travelled anywhere outside my comfort zone. Up until then, I'd been taken to French hotels in Cap d'Antibes with blue-and-white-striped umbrellas lined up along the shoreline. Wearing just bikini bottoms, I'd gone on pedaloes with my parents and caught crabs in buckets. I'd lain in the sand, damp with salt and seawater, and waited for the sun-kissed vendors to come roaming down the beachfront in their Speedos, selling tepid bottles of Orangina and packets of hot, sugar-coated, crunchy peanuts. I'd stayed in swanky hotel rooms, with whirring white fans over-head, and listened to the buzz of mosquitoes at night as my baby sister slept in a cot beside me, her plump little legs dangling through the bars. I'd breakfasted on white peaches and grappled with elegant cubes of butter that nestled in bowls of ice cubes, ready to melt into crumbly croissants.

I'd gone to California and stayed at the Beverly Hills Hotel. When jet lag kicked in at 3 a.m., my sister and I would switch on the telly in our room and watch *Looney Tunes* cartoons on a loop, before switching over to *I Love Lucy* as the peachy dawn rose outside our window. We greeted the new day square-eyed and delirious with excitement and lack of sleep.

We'd sometimes dress alike (despite our six-year age gap) in Danskin shorts and T-shirts; our hair tightly ponytailed or in bunches. We'd breakfast at The Soda Fountain and order crispy bacon and waffles or neon-coloured Froot Loops, before running down to the pool. Our base was our cabana, a shady sanctuary full of freshly folded towels and iced water. We'd swim for hours – holding our breath, turning cartwheels, racing each other, diving for coins, doing lengths, mucking about. Coming out for lunch, shrivelled and dehydrated, ravenous for burgers and fries and plea-bargaining with our parents for a Sprite. Golden days.

I try to tell the doctor that Jordan blew my mind. I'd never been to a country that had armed soldiers at the airport, and dusty roads full of tanks and old Mercedes. I'd never looked at a menu and not really known what I wanted to eat. Nor had I ever stayed in one of those municipal beige hotels that were lacking in charm but full of marble. But equally I'd never been anywhere as exotic and as magnificent as Petra.

It is this aspect I choose to talk to my Jordanian doctor about as he preps my skin with iodine.

'Very good,' he says as he goes in. 'Nice. I'm getting lovely samples.'

I stop talking about Petra and take myself off to the ceiling.

'Is it normal to feel . . .' I bleat. 'Is it normal to feel heat and tingling and . . . pain?'

'It's okay, my dear,' says my Placater, gripping my flailing hand tightly. 'You are doing very well.'

'All done,' says the doctor, finally. 'All good. You were very brave.'

I am shaking. 'I don't think I was brave,' I say apologetically, my lip indented with teeth marks, my hand still clawed into a fist.

'Most men cry,' he replies. 'Women are brave.'

Buoyed up by my genetic disposition and the fact I have survived, I ask to see what little bit of my body they've removed this time.

He proudly holds up a tiny glass jar with what looks like bloodied dead worms. Pink squiggles. The bush-tucker trial is over. I've won dinner for my camp.

Relief.

Back at home, Johnnie and I metaphorically cross off the days on the calendar, and I worry about Archie. There's another drama taking place in his life, no less pressing, which is running parallel to mine.

Archie has a chocolate-brown Labrador called Hank. Johnnie and I bought Hank for him seven years ago, when Arch was living alone and worryingly miserable. I thought having something to love and care for might make him happier. Emotional support. And, as it turned out, Hank has made everyone happy; not just Archie. He is one of the family. I used to call him my first grandchild. My furry grand-dog. I love him passionately, and if ever Archie goes away, I kidnap his dog. We are close. I give him bits of cheese and let him sleep on my bed, and I tickle his tummy as I'm falling asleep.

But Hank has developed a weird limp. Amid all my medical dramas, Archie has been dealing with vet's appointments. First they did blood tests, then a biopsy of his lymph nodes. Now Archie is trailing after him every morning, collecting urine samples in order for them to ascertain if his kidneys are okay. Hank is almost mirroring my symptoms. It's as if one of us has Munchausen's syndrome. How is this even possible? Like those dogs currently being trained to sniff out Covid, has Hank already developed some sort of canine psychic ability because we are so close?

I can't bear it. I can't bear anything to be wrong with Hanky. Not now. We need him. We all need him. Archie really needs him.

Archie has already had to go beyond the call of filial duty. He was the one who drove to Bethnal Green on Tilly's birthday and told her I had cancer. He was the one who went to his grandmother's and sat on the sofa, making tiny talk, before bursting into tears and telling her the news. It broke my heart that he'd do that for me. We need Hank to not limp and to stop peeing excessively and to be here for all of us. Especially Archie.

My entire family is working overtime to make light of what is happening. We don't ignore it. But we are all massively pretending, in that slightly verging-on-hysterical British way, that everything is going to be just fine. Dandy. It's a piece of cake. A blip. I'm trying my best to lead by example. I'm keeping it bright and breezy for my kids, my mum, my sister, Johnnie. I feel voicing fear is almost more infectious than this godforsaken pandemic, and I have a great desire to infect my family only with optimism. I'm going to play the part of Little Miss Optimistic to the best of my ability. It's terribly important to me.

We're a theatrical family, prone to being overdramatic. Emotions could easily escalate, unless I rein them in. We're all good at acting. And don't forget, I've actively decided not to google anything. Not to ask for statistics, or survival rates. I've turned that part of my normally inquisitive, journalistic brain off at the mains. Flicked the switch. All I am certain of is that I am going to give it everything I have in me, in order not to end up as a name spoken in memoriam, or as a fading photograph gathering dust on the bedside table of those I love the most. It doesn't occur to me that my poor family might lack my willpower.

It is only later that I realise they are having to cope with this poisoned chalice behind my back. Six separate households only talking about how they feel whenever I am out of earshot. I am the elephant in the room. We aren't facing up to this collectively, but individually. Johnnie. My mum. My sister in America. India, Huck and Sean. Archie, Nisha and Billy. Tilly.

I think I've created this isolation because I feel the need to keep a tight hold on my vulnerability, my terror. I've never liked appearing exposed or needy. I pretend everything is under control; in order to control myself. A cancer diagnosis and Covid. And another fucking lockdown.

Life is handing out a lot of lemons, and I am still trying to make lemonade. Bitter-sweet lemonade.

Finally, it's the day of the Big Reveal. C-Day. It's a Tuesday night. Johnnie thinks the traffic will be bad getting to Harley Street so orders a taxi far, far too early. I don't want to be early, so am petulant and ungrateful. He talks to the taxi driver about bicycle lanes and traffic cones and the Mayor of London. I sit with my forehead against the window, watching the rain, as we zoom down Park Lane at dusk.

Archie is already waiting outside the doctor's office for us, and we shuffle in like three silent, masked Musketeers. The seats in the waiting room are sixties lime green, and we socially distance. We're very early. Obviously. I can hear the doctor in his office talking to another patient.

Six o'clock comes and goes.

Six fifteen.

I am jiggling. I am rubbing my hands up and down my trousers.

I go to the loo.

Archie goes to the loo.

Johnnie tries to engage both of us in a painting of Egyptian temples hanging on the opposite wall and gives us a mini lecture on ancient history.

I'm not listening. I am incapable of concentrating.

I go to pee again.

I stare ahead.

The doctor's door flies open.

'Sorry, sorry. Sorry to keep you waiting. I appreciate it. I know I'm running late, but I have a slight problem with the patient I'm seeing. If it's any consolation, I've got all your reports in and it's all good news. Exactly as I thought initially. Bear with me for another ten minutes.' The doctor rushes back to his office.

I burst into uncontrollable, convulsive, heaving, snotty tears. I crumble in on myself. 'Oh my God,' I gasp. 'I think I'm going to be okay. Perhaps I'm not going to die. It's not a space invader. It's not a spreader. I can get better.' I'm rocking backwards and forwards, repeating myself.

Gulping down life. Pushing my immortality back to first base. 'I just didn't want to leave any of you.'

'Mum, Mum,' says Archie, pulling off his mask, tears streaming down his face, and enveloping my shaking body with his arms. 'I always knew you were going to be okay,' he says, before adding a black-humoured aside. 'Honestly, this week I've been more worried about Hank than you. I always knew *you* were going to be all right.'

I sniffle and smile.

One for all, and all for one, I think to myself, as we all troop into the office, Johnnie squeezing my hand so tightly in support that it goes deliciously numb.

Archie records the conversation and later plays it back to the rest of the family, all of whom are collectively relieved. With the right course of hard-core treatment, the odds are high I will beat this.

Who ever knew bad news could be so good?

Long, long after I've finished chemo and am a year into my maintenance programme, I realise I didn't take in or remember a single word the doctor told me that day.

Not one.

I do recall being there, but I must, subconsciously, have eradicated all references to the Grade 3 tumour and the highly descriptive 'aggressive' adjective that was flung about. I obviously nuked that information the second it attempted to find a neural pathway into my brain.

So I remain blissfully (or perhaps stubbornly) oblivious to the medical severity of my situation. Until fourteen months later, when my post-chemo PET scan comes back clear. I accept that I've been up shit creek, but I must have put myself into a self-survival trance of denial.

Meanwhile, my poor family carried the heavy burden of knowledge.

I find it hard to forgive myself for that. It was supremely selfish of me.

I must now filter the updates back to my darling mum – carefully, because of her Peter Pan attitude to illness. She who has always convinced me I could do anything I ever wanted to in life, she who has filled me with confidence and optimism, is doing what any mother worth her salt would do. She's trying to make it better. Put a good spin on the ordeal that awaits me.

'I somehow don't think you will lose your hair,' she tells me, with confidence. 'I have a strong hunch you will be one of those people who keep theirs.' No one can polish a turd quite like my mum. 'You will probably sail through chemo and be one of those people who don't feel sick.'

The problem is, Mummy, I'm not special. I'm not special any more. I'm broken. You alone can't make me better, nor can you make this hurt go away.

And that's an odd realisation for a child to have to acknowledge. My mother has always – like me – seen her cup as being half full. She was (and still is) a proper low-maintenance, natural beauty. No expensive time-consuming tweaks, treatments and medical improvements for my mum. She genuinely never needed them. I could sense she was glamourous – even when I was too young to understand what the word actually meant.

She has always, always had my back. An only child whose both parents were touring vaudevillians, she had a peripatetic childhood. Money was always tight. And from what she's told me, although she had a lot of love, stability and nurturing, it was a necessarily abstemious upbringing, with the few toys she owned sometimes sold to make ends meet.

She brought Emma and me up to appreciate everything we had. To turn any small event into a grand occasion. To have the ability to go both upmarket and down and get the same enjoyment from both experiences. Woolworths and Harrods. Bournemouth and Hollywood. Peanut butter sandwiches and steak. I am so grateful she instilled this lust for life – all of it – in me; never taking anything for granted, always appreciating every small detail, and never placing a monetary value on pleasures.

She was a hands-on mother, insisting on good manners and routine, and she loved encouraging us to be creative. Endless crafts and colouring, make-believe and fantasy games. One Easter, she popped a tiny live chick inside a cardboard egg and hid it in the garden for me to find. She'd let me concoct revolting cocktails (Ribena, milk and rotting petals from the garden) and offer them to dinner guests, without making fun of my early entertaining efforts. She'd help me make endless pretend newspapers, which I'd laboriously work on; interviewing my friends and cutting bits out of magazines and making collages.

She let me decorate my bedroom myself when I became a teenager, and she was forever the 'welcoming' mum who never said no to friends coming over for tea and sleepovers.

Once, when I was being truculent and bolshy (and quite possibly rude as well), she told me that she would always, always love me, no matter what I did, but today she was finding it hard to actually like me. Fair cop.

Although she periodically worked throughout my childhood, as both an actress and children's author, she never failed to put us first. I wear Fracas to this day because it's like being embraced by her. The smell reminds me of being tucked into bed at night as a child, and I will forever associate it with the security and love in which she enveloped me. I drench myself with it now I am sick and unable to physically see her. Just as Noël Coward observed the potency of cheap music, I subliminally recognise the transformative powers of familiarity sprayed on a broken body.

The year after my dad died, Elton John invited my mum and me to Las Vegas, to see him perform at Caesars Palace. As his guests. A massive treat.

Elton came into our lives when I was twelve; turning up at the bookshop my dad owned in Virginia Water, in platform shoes and dyed green hair. Initially, my dad mistook him for one of the Bee Gees, who lived nearby, but after discovering he was 'another' pop star, Elton became a close, close family friend. The son my dad never had. Elton is an insanely generous, thoughtful, kind man and one of those rare human beings who never demands gratitude. He just loves being able to share his good fortune, and enjoys seeing his friends bask in the pleasures he's made possible.

So off we went to Viva Las Vegas, for five days. It was the first time I can recall us ever going on a trip together. Just the two of us. I've travelled a lot on my own. My mum less so. If at all, in living memory. My dad always took the controls, and now I was assuming his role. Tickets. Passports. Security. It was a bit like travelling with a chic, immaculately dressed child. And I, her companion, was dressed in mufti, attempting to get her to follow the multitudinous rules.

She did needlepoint on the long flight, and slept. Upright. I binge-watched movies, spilt a cup of coffee down my sweatshirt, and remained wide awake throughout. My mother looked stunning as we disembarked. Fresh. She'd applied a deft slick of lipstick and had backcombed her hair in the loo. I looked crumpled and covered in crumbs.

I love the shameless vulgarity of Vegas. The round-the-clock 'awakeness' of the place. It's the dream location for an insomniac. You lose track of time as you wander through the labyrinths of gaming rooms, corridors and blinged-up stores selling endless branded merchandise.

We had adjoining suites, with the equivalent of an extremely overpriced corner shop as well as a minibar the size of a village off-licence. Our 'shop' was stacked with jars of nuts, chocolates, disposable cameras, guidebooks, cookies, crisps, plastic-tasting American muffins. And condoms. We were in Vegas, after all. Of course there were condoms.

Unbeknownst to me, whenever my mother woke early with jet lag, she would rearrange the shelves. Make them look prettier. My mum makes everything look better. More attractive. It's an innate skill she must have been born with; creating little tableaux of prettiness. Each one a still life. So she'd line up the jars of nuts. Examine the cameras. Flick through the guidebooks. Eat a chocolate or two.

We behaved like teenagers. We hung out together. We watched crap TV. Read magazines. Ripped out recipes to try out when we got home. Ate unhealthy food. Snacked. Got coffee from Starbucks – which was downstairs, in the hotel lobby. We went shopping in ridiculous shops called Forever 21, and bought ridiculous clothes that looked vaguely right in Vegas, but monstrous as soon as we got back home. We trawled drugstores and tried on different lipsticks and blushers. We fed quarters into the slot machines for ten minutes at a time; limiting the inevitable losses. And stared, open mouthed, at the ashen-faced gamblers who stayed glued to their seats for hours in that airless, unreal atmosphere. We laughed a lot.

We met Elton for lunch every day and had fries with everything. We saw his show. Twice. It was electrifying. We boogied whilst balancing paper cups filled with luke-warm white wine. He sang all the oldies: 'Crocodile Rock', 'Rocket Man', 'Your Song'. He dedicated 'Don't Let the Sun Go Down on Me' to my dad. He said Daddy had changed his life. Mum and I both cried. Happy-sad tears. We went to Cirque du Soleil, to the Michael Jackson show, and saw a strange magician do amazing tricks.

When it came time to check out and go home, I went downstairs to settle the bill. Despite the fact that Elton was adamant we were his guests, and had given us firm instructions we were to pay for nothing, I was determined to cover the internet, breakfasts in bed, movies we'd watched and the minibar we'd plundered.

'I'd like to settle the bill for Nanette Forbes and Sarah Standing, please.'

'Certainly, madam. Right. Your extras for room 1123 are $210, and the bill for Mrs Forbes, in 1124, is $2,425.'

I stood at reception, aghast. What on earth had my mother charged to her room?

'Right,' I said. 'Could I possibly just check her bill?'

The cashier printed it off the screen and handed it to me across the desk.

1 jar of cashews	$22
2 Diet Cokes	$12
4 bottles of water	$20
4 breakfasts	$245 (excluding taxes & service)
2 movies	$24
3 bars of chocolate	$36
And about a million condoms	!!!

'I think there must be some mistake. My mother is eighty-three, newly widowed, and there is no way she could – or indeed would – ever buy condoms. Could you be really sweet and double-check there hasn't been some mistake?'

'No, ma'am, there is no mistake.'

'But there must be,' I implored.

'All our room items are electronically tagged. You pick them up and they automatically get added to your bill,' the cashier explained, rather tersely.

Ah. The rearranging. The creating pretty tableaux. The biding time at the crack of dawn before I woke up. The fiddling with the corner shop's wares. It all suddenly made sense. My darling mum had effectively bought hundreds of contraceptives. Enough condoms to supply a large fraternity house. God bless her.

They removed the condoms from the bill, after a fair bit of persuasion. I know that what happens in Vegas is supposed to stay in Vegas.

But not this story.

Elton and his husband, David, become my saviours during lockdown, chemo and Covid. They make my mother part of their bubble and take unbelievable care of her. Inviting her to lunch every Sunday, once restrictions become slightly more fluid; checking up on her every day.

She has shoulders to cry on, belonging to two men who truly love her.

Their care and their calming reassurance make our forced separation bearable. For both of us.

4

Daily life speeds by. I go for a walk in Battersea Park with India and Huck. Fresh air feels safe. We meet up with Archie and Nisha and baby Billy. It's the most stunning late-autumnal morning. Bright and crisp and sunny. The park is rammed. I'm so happy to be with both my grandsons, two of my children, and Hank. I've temporarily managed to put everything negative out of my mind during this walk, and I'm high-octane happy. I'm seeing rainbows where there are none.

It's such a perfect day. We bump into Anya and sip coffees by the lake, and the sunlight hits our collective highlights and bathes us in golden hues. Billy laughs in his pushchair and I get him out and snuggle him. Huck holds my hand.

We all take a glut of photographs.

Instagram them.

#SmileyHappyPeople.

Family. My everything.

Freeze-frame.

And now it's time for chemo. Round one.

I'm coming at this bugger like Captain Hook. Sword out, ready to slay. And I'm not interested in Neverland. I genuinely don't need reassurance – I'm too much of a realist. I'm feeling much too bitter to swallow any pill that's been sugar coated.

I go into hospital to meet my chemo team. More bloods. More Covid tests. I try to put my house in order. I redo a page of wishes, to go alongside my will, but succeed in making myself cry so much I have to stop and abort the exercise altogether. Put it on the back burner. I can't go there just now. I can't think of anything. I'm robotic. On autopilot. Going through the motions, blotting out emotions. I pay bills and set up a weekly Ocado delivery. I clear out cupboards with manic energy. Circling, circling, circling. I feel like a hawk that has spied a little field mouse scuttling in the long grass below him. I'm just waiting to dive.

I talk to positive friends who've come out the other side. Louise Fennell, one of my oldest friends, is incredible. She's been there, got the T-shirt, and is living proof that family, friends and sick humour are what get you through. When she was diagnosed with breast cancer, two decades ago, she made me promise her one thing. We were on our way to visit a shop called Lunn Antiques, to stock up on pretty nighties for her to wear in hospital post-op.

'If I don't make it, you've got to somehow intercept my Peter Jones card,' she urged me. 'Theo has simply no idea how much I've managed to run up on it. Promise me you'll just tell them to jump for it? Write them a letter and inform them I've emigrated to Australia – or snuffed it. Be brutal.'

I don't think I've ever loved Louise more than at that moment. I just knew for certain she was going to live to settle those frigging minimum payments. She had the right attitude.

I'm trying to channel Louise's positivity now. Making light of the situation. Today I'm dressed in black. Head to toe. Tilly comes over and is also dressed in black. We both look like depressed characters from a Chekhov play.

'Snap,' I say. 'We're in mourning for my life.'

We laugh too loudly and high-five each other, without actually touching. Covid might catch us.

'Like Nina from *The Seagull*,' I say.

Black humour.

They say, as a parent, you are only ever as happy as your unhappiest child. Possibly the biggest silver lining I'm looking at right now is the fact that Tilly is happy. She's in love with a totally delightful young man called Felix Archer, and her joy is infectious. It lights up a room. She's like a glow-worm. She's not relying on me for emotional support, she's chucked the maternal crutch and has stopped hobbling. She's found someone sensational. Same values, same sort of family; he fits like a glove. And I can tell he simply adores her. And what's more, he professes to genuinely love Abba; potentially on a par with me. The winner indeed takes it all. They'd only been seeing each other for about six weeks before I fired a bullet into Tilly's heart.

'You don't have to stick around for this,' Tilly told him. 'It's going to get hairy.'

Felix's reply was immediate. 'I'm not going anywhere. I'm in. The walks are just going to get longer, the coffee stronger and the hugs more frequent.' He nailed his flag to the mast, without hesitation. A true keeper.

But bloody hell. Cancer is the gift you can't hand back.

Prior to my first chemo session I have to have a port fitted. 'Fitted' is another medical euphemism. I get bathrooms fitted, contraceptive coils fitted, carpets fitted. Surely you don't get a semi-permanent catheter inserted under your clavicle, right by your jugular, *fitted*? The very thought shrivels my front bottom.

I'm given a book called *Understanding Chemotherapy* and another called something like *Caring for Your Port*, and I don't even open them. I leave the hospital and dump them in the nearest bin. I'm halfway through reading Barbara Amiel's *Friends and Enemies*, which is a book I can dip in and out of and is much more my cup of tea than medical instruction manuals. I have decided that what I don't medically swot up on, time will reveal regardless. Understanding chemo isn't going to make me like it more, or tolerate it better. And I'm never going to care for my own port. Nor am I going to let Johnnie anywhere near it with slightly shaky eighty-six-year-old hands. Or snatchy, grabby Billy aged nine months. My port is going to remain undercover, hidden from sight, and tended to only by professionals. No self-care for me.

To have the port fitted, I get to go under. I have my first general anaesthetic ever. Three weeks ago, I'd have been terrified at the thought of having one, now I'm pitifully grateful not to have it done with a local. I've had enough done to me already, with nothing to numb the pain except my own fingernails digging into my palm. I feel like I've been upgraded from Economy to First Class. I've turned left. No more 'simple procedures' for me, I'm in with the big boys. I'm going under the knife.

An extremely nervous Filipino student nurse appears at the bottom of my bed and explains he was a nurse ten years ago, but then returned to the Philippines, set up a business that failed, and is now back training again. Is it okay if he asks me some important questions?

'Of course,' I reply.

'Are you pregnant?'

'Sorry?'

'Might you be pregnant?'

'I am sixty-one years old,' I say, very slowly.

'Then can you remember the date of your last period?'

'Mercifully not, no. I can't.'

Student nurse laboriously writes down this information.

'Can I help you with anything else, madam?'

'My surgical stockings?' I say.

He deftly uncurls the stockings, sliding them up my legs, like the reverse skinning of a snake.

I lie in my room, waiting to be taken down to theatre. My body is covered with one of those stiff, white blankets with holes, the sheet endlessly rucking up and annoying me.

And we're off!

Off on one of those weird journeys, down a labyrinth of hospital corridors and through flapping doors, where you're lying flat on your back clocking cracks in the ceiling, counting the fluorescent lights rushing overhead, gliding past mirrored lifts and distorted faces.

A friend has told me that I'll love being put under. She said it's like gulping down a second gin and tonic. Even though I don't drink gin, I am sort of looking forward to the experience.

Not that I can really say I experienced it. After my corridor adventure, I find myself mid-conversation in a side room with three nurses who are getting ready to go home for the night.

The clock opposite me says it is 10 p.m. It is very quiet.

'Do you have far to go?' I ask.

'Claire does,' replies her male colleague. 'She lives near Forest Gate.'

'Roughly what time do you think I will have the operation?' I ask, aware of the fact my throat is savagely dry.

'It's done, my darling,' cackles the third nurse. 'You are good to go. It's over. Done.'

'You're kidding me?' I say.

And then I look down at my newly acquired accessories. I appear to have a blue dishcloth stuck down to my upper chest with a transparent plaster. A white dressing on my jugular, and a hanging ornament – known as a 'gripper'. A gripper is where they attach the tube that the chemo will go through tomorrow. I am indeed good to go.

My front bottom contracts. This shit show just got real.

The following morning, I having stayed overnight in hospital recovering from my mini-op, the chemo arrives in its own bag.

I'm staggered it didn't come complete with security guards. It's in one of those insulated containers one normally takes on summer picnics. It looks as if it should be full of carrot sticks and hummus, resting on one of those slightly musty-smelling ice packs. Enter R-CHOP aka 'the Red Devil'. Its nickname is the Red Devil. No shit. It's like liquid neon. It's a fluorescent, mind-expanding orange colour and in a syringe the size of a bottle of Lucozade. It looks fake. Like a bad prop from a B movie.

Maria comes with it. Maria is big and loud and lovely. Jolly.

'Baby girl, you and I are going to do this together. I'm not leaving your side until this is all gone. It's going to be okay, cos I'm here with you.'

My eyes prick with tears. She's so kind. All the nurses are so kind.

'You ever been to Zimbabwe?' she asks as she flushes my port and fiddles about with my gripper.

'No,' I reply. 'I've been all over India but never Africa. I'd like to one day.'

Slight lie. I've never held the faintest desire to go to Africa, but I am totally committed to sitting here with my gripper out, clutching Maria's hand for support. Listening to her stories of zebras and hippos, and exotic dishes made with ground beef and rice, whilst being injected with something so toxic it makes Monster Munch look like a health food.

And then it's over.

Done.

More drips put in and flushed. And bags of anti-nausea liquid hung up. And immune-boosting stuff pumped in. And infusions.

And I'm left alone.

I shuffle off to the loo. I immediately pee toxic-coloured urine. I imagine my tumour being blasted out of its hiding place. Imploded. Unsettled. Take that, you fuckpig. I'm attacking you with an Uzi and you are going to end up the loser.

I'm euphoric. One down, five to go. And I feel nothing except relief.

I watch telly from my hospital bed and telephone my family and friends. And try to ignore the blue dishcloth attached to my breastbone, and the bandage attached to my neck, and the post-operative tenderness.

A massive gift is delivered to my room. It's from Anya

Hindmarch. Anya is a close neighbour and, despite having five children, a husband and an empire to run, is one of those women who somehow always finds the time to be an amazing friend. One of those rare ones you'd throb to go into the jungle with. She's stalwart, steady and wise. I can't even remember how we first met, but I'm eternally grateful we did.

My present is a custom-made, newly christened 'chemo bag', chic as hell, packed to the gills with everything anyone going through what I'm going through alone could ever wish for. Labelled pockets for glasses, coins, earphones, water, hand sanitiser. Compartments for a laptop and books, and spare knickers and pens. She's stuffed it with the most thoughtful things: dark-coloured nail varnishes for when my nails turn that deadly yellow; Polo mints for my dry mouth; a selection of magazines; a mini bottle of vodka for party times; a monogrammed leather folder to encourage me to keep writing this book; a silky, stuffed-toy chocolate-brown Labrador. I mean, who runs a highly successful business and manages to find a stuffed chocolate-brown Labrador during lockdown?

And there's a note. And the note destroys me. It is beyond loving.

I think it's the first time I've allowed myself the luxury of a really good, cathartic cry. A cry that is uninterrupted. Not overheard. Volatile. One that eventually sends me to sleep with snail trails of tears staining my cheeks.

But not for long.

At about 2 a.m., I wake up with the frigging Uzi pointed up against my temple. I have sap rising in my head. I'm on fire. The sap's bubbling like the witches' cauldron in *Macbeth*. It's not like a headache or a migraine, this is a different kettle of fish altogether. I'm sweating. I push the buzzer for help.

The night nurse comes in and takes my blood pressure and tests my oxygen levels. They're low. She makes me sit up and drink water and reassures me this is normal. She gives me two paracetamol. Hospitals give you paracetamol for literally *everything*, I've come to realise: it's their go-to drug.

I momentarily settle down. But it's short-lived.

An hour later, I'm on the floor in the bathroom, dry retching. Sweating. Feeble. Wasted. Unable to get up. Head swirling. Get this fucking Uzi out of my face!

I pull the stringy little red emergency buzzer next to the loo. I'm lying like a beetle; needy as fuck. Help me. This can't be normal.

Two nurses gently get me back to bed and give me more anti-nausea meds.

It's 4 a.m. I watch *The Queen's Gambit* on my laptop until dawn.

The Red Devil has made its presence known.

Game on.

Port out. Starboard home.

60

5

Johnnie has made my bed plump and cosy, and filled my bedside table with bottles of water and Ritz crackers and pears. I'm on steroids. Big steroids.

Steroids make me feel utterly fabulous. It's time-travelling back to the eighties of my misspent youth. It's going on a five-day bender and clubbing every night. It's like sniffing cocaine and knocking back tequila shots and dancing manically to Donna Summer and the Village People for hours on end. It's flirting with the waiters at Studio 54 in their minuscule satin shorts, and going into back rooms in the basement, and gurning with strangers and jigging on bar stools. It's squinting to greet the dawn, stinking of cigarettes, with sticky feet and clammy hands. Steroids are the feel-good prize you get when you've completed a round of chemo.

Sleep is for wimps when I'm on steroids. Too much to do. Too much clearing out of cupboards, too much cooking, too much talking. It's heaven. The false energy and sense of well-being is off the charts. It's like being seventeen years old again. Reliving those glory, Duracell Bunny days, when nights had no clocks.

A month ago, Johnnie bought Tilly a second-hand car as an early birthday and Christmas present. She's collecting it tonight from the garage down the road and is going to do a drive past. At thirty-one she's waited a long time to have wheels. We've planned to have a socially distanced, masked show-and-tell.

Up she rolls. Parallel parks (perfectly) across the road. We go out and admire it from afar. It's dusk.

Johnnie and I aren't really admiring the car, we're actually basking in the transformation of our youngest daughter. Her happiness. She's on fire with joy. She puts on a CD and cranks up the volume. She gets out of the car and performs karaoke to an imaginary microphone.

Suddenly, we are all three of us dancing with abandon on the pavement. Far apart but close. The light from the street lamp casts shadows, and from further down the road, three fabulously elegant young Black men join us. Their bodies sway to the music. And although we are all masked, I can tell they are grinning. Two small children appear at a window, and their mother opens it to see what all the fuss is about. Now they too are clapping to the music. Tilly's boyfriend, Felix, appears in an Uber, to drive home with her. They hug. This is living. This is a true magic moment. This is what life is all about.

I will treasure it forever. Truly. It is totally perfect.

*

I'm starting to create a new normal.

Too nervous to shower, for fear of getting my port wet, I bathe and then lean over the side of the bath to wash my hair separately. My hair. My glorious hair. No rubbing, no rough play. Gentle strokes, from top to bottom. A little conditioner. Washing in tepid water. No brushing. I'm too scared to brush, so my hair is wild and untamed. I sleep on special spunky pillowcases that the hospital has recommended. White silk-satin. Playboy Mansion, bunny-girl pillowcases. They're slimy and slippery, and vaguely revolting, but apparently protect the hair. I just wish my hair could have a twenty-four-hour bodyguard of its very own. It needs all the protection I can possibly afford.

On my many pre-chemo, early-morning walks with Anya around Battersea Park, we had a rhythm. Rules. Strict rules. We took turns running through the trials of our everyday lives. A checklist. Kids, husbands, work, parents. In that order. During the first lockdown, Anya wrote a book; a light-hearted, astute, self-help manual on life, family and business. We used to stride around the park discussing titles, and now it's ended up being called *If in Doubt, Wash Your Hair*. Brilliant title. How totally ironic that I am now terrified of doing exactly that. I know it's going to go. I'm not brave enough to pre-empt the inevitable. It's my mane. I've never had short hair in my life. And obviously, I've never been bald. I've ordered a bespoke wig, and I joke about it, but I don't find it funny. I think the day my hair falls out will be the day I crash down off the ceiling and have a reality check.

Meanwhile, my steroid honeymoon comes to an end. I leave Studio 54, still a fraction high and buoyed up, and try to get on with everyday life. But wait. I forgot there was a nasty little bully lurking in the playground. A snarling pit bull. A character Vinnie Jones might play; a menacing little scumbag that waits to leap out at me and attack. His name is Chemo.

Chemo likes to insidiously send a tsunami through my body and beat the shit out of me when I least expect it. And I'm a novice, lest we forget.

Gums: sore, fuzzy.

Teeth relentlessly coated in a scuzzy film.

Metallic taste like crunching tinfoil.

Eyes: flickering, going in and out of focus.

Bowels: not functioning.

Lower back: agony. A deep, deep pain that is constant. Standing up, lying down.

The Chemo bully boy has floored me with this one. He's throwing left hooks and pounding me with pain.

'Thought you could handle the Red Devil, did you? You little piece of shit. No one fucks with the Red Devil and comes out unscathed,' the bully boy announces, pushing me up against the wall with a mocking sneer of victory.

I stumble to my feet and call the twenty-four-hour helpline at the hospital.

'It's totally normal,' they reassure me. 'It's coming from your bones and is a side effect of the medicine we gave you, strapped to your arm, when you left the hospital. Take paracetamol. It will go.'

That night, Johnnie checks up on me every two hours. He's worried. Feels helpless. 'What can I do?' he asks, gently stroking my head.

He's panicking, I can tell. I've never really been ill before. Nor have I put him in a position where he's had to take medical decisions on my behalf, beyond fetching me a hot-water bottle or migraine pills. His fear is palpable and makes me feel sad. This has got to be just as hard on him as it is on me.

'Should I take you back to hospital? What do you want me to do? What can I do? Tell me, sweetheart. I'll do anything. Anything. Just say, and I'll do it. What do you think is causing this pain?'

'Cancer,' I whimper. 'It's the chemo. And the cancer. The medicines. If you take me to hospital at this stage of the game, I'm scared I will never come home. I'm going to have to get used to it, I guess. I'll be okay tomorrow.'

He lies beside me and strokes my head until I fall asleep.

And two days later, the pain goes. The Chemo bully boy gets bored and slinks off for a few days.

My teeth stop feeling quite so fuzzy. I feel hungry for the first time in weeks. I devour Marmite on toast, and spinach rolls studded with nuggets of feta cheese.

No dairy. Have to avoid dairy – and boy do I love dairy. But I'm allowed to eat feta. I grow to love feta. Feta is my saviour.

I now have two of my oldest friends going through cancer treatment. Different types, but we are united and in constant contact. We make one another laugh, we compare drugs, we have a newfound, easy shorthand.

Milica is the Don. I rang her from my hospital bed the night I was first diagnosed, alone and terrified.

'I've gone and joined your bloody stupid club, Mil. It's not all about you any more. I've become a life member and you're going to have to show me the ropes.'

She's got two Stage 4 cancers and is extraordinary and inspirational in her fortitude, bravery and humour. We talk at five in the morning, when we are both wide awake, and text at night when insomnia hits. She's like family to me. I've known her since the day she was born (because our mothers were great friends), and I used to play with her three older brothers. Indeed, I went out with her brother Cassian, and we babysat Mil sometimes and picked her up from school. We lived close to one another as kids, and although Milica is much younger than I, we have remained close. We share the shorthand of childhood.

That first night, I felt like an imposter beside her – she's the real deal, and I'm just a little wannabe.

But Mil is bigger than that, and generous. She figuratively holds my hand on FaceTime. And I hope I sometimes talk her off the ledge of unreason on the rare occasions she feels like throwing the towel in.

Ben has cancer of the blood, and he's sanguine and funny and bitter. He's a film and television director; he and his wife Jo were practically the first people Johnnie introduced me to when we began dating. Ben and I mainly laugh about the bitterness we feel towards the deck of cards we've been dealt. We used to talk about movies and actors and the time we all lived in Los Angeles together. Now we talk about the 'entry-level dose for codeine' and 'low platelet count' and 'oral chemo as opposed to intra-venous', and then we both get bored and just amuse each other and wish we could stop shielding and actually meet up in person.

It's funny the little things that get you through the days and nights. My sister picked two stones up off the beach when I was first diagnosed. White, smooth, oval stones. She wrote on them 'you' and 'me' and drew little smiley faces. They come everywhere with me. My talis-mans. More precious than diamonds.

My friends Victoria and Emma came and replanted the pots outside my front door with winter plants and flowers. Puffed up against the cold in Uniqlo jackets, with a bag of compost in the boot of their car, they worked tirelessly to make it all look festive and beautiful. And alive. The alive bit is important. I often open my front door to just gaze at my pots, slowly drinking in the winter beauty of cyclamens and those feathery, frosted, silver ferns that look like they belong under the ocean.

My brother-in-law finds a celebrity website that en-ables you to pay a variety of celebs to record special, personalised messages. He goes big. No John Cleese wishing me a happy birthday for $50, he pulls out the big bucks and gets Caitlin Jenner to talk to me for a full five minutes.

'Sarah, Caitlyn Jenner here. Now I've had to face a lot of adversity in my life, and one just has to be determined. I understand you are going through rough times at the moment, but you will get through this. You have a great family, and they are all here for you. Graham reached out to me, told me your story, and although he can't be with you physically, he is right by your side.'

It's the most original pick-me-up – and funny as hell.

India plays Word Hunt on GamePigeon with me. It's a game of anagrams we can play against each other on our phones. Ind tends to keep her emotions under wraps, but this game has become like our private SOS. A 999 call. When my phone pings, requesting a game, I know she's got me in her thoughts. In hospital, when I felt wretched and sick, she didn't give up.

Ping.

Play with me, Mum, I'm here. You aren't alone.

Ping.

Keep going. Don't give up.

Ping.

Beat me. Beat cancer.

She wins every time, but I fully intend to whip her ass.

Tilly comes and stands outside our front door most days. An extremely welcome and mini visitation. Often with a cup of coffee. I think she needs physical proof that I'm still standing. Which I can't actually do for any prolonged length of time before I start to feel woozy.

Archie calls me. Sleep deprived from broken baby nights, he checks in regularly, but I can sense he's too traumatised to fully engage in the reality of what's happening to me. He self-protects by skirting around the issue, and concentrates just on the practicalities. 'When is your next appointment, Mum?' He subconsciously asks only those questions that bypass feelings, and then steers our conversations towards safer, shallower waters. We talk about Billy's first tooth, or the fact he loves sweet potatoes. And I understand. I get it.

If we both pretend this isn't happening, perhaps we can make-believe it isn't real.

I have a deep, plum-coloured bruise on my wrist that my watch doesn't hide. It reminds me of my father Bryan Forbes who died six years ago, and I hate it for that reason. It reminds me of death. It's where the cannula goes in, and always leaves its mark. During the last three years of his life, his withered arms were speckled with blood bruises.

I'm glad my dad isn't around to see me go through this. He wasn't good with illness or pain. His or anyone else's. To him, hospitals were fearful places. Places you went to die, not get better. Born in 1926, twenty-two years before the NHS was founded, I guess he had good reason. He was the most faultless father a girl could wish for, and I loved him passionately. He was fiercely intelligent and inquisitive; well read and self-educated and self-aware. He kept a detailed journal throughout his life. He was brave during the war. He faced professional adversity with dignity and aplomb, yet was curiously constipated when it came to any disease. He couldn't do blood or gore. He had a childlike terror of all routine hospital procedures. Blood tests, transfusions, MRI scans, X-rays: he was wary of all of them. He used to make my sister go with him and put on a lead coat when he was wheeled off for an X-ray; it scared him so.

Daddy wouldn't have known what to do with me. The word 'cancer' would have thrown him off the cliff of reason. He could (and did) write about extreme experiences, and he directed scenes in movies where the heroine died; but he was incapable of addressing these huge emotions in real life.

Although I never stopped thinking he would. I kept praying if I got him alone towards the end of his life, he'd hold my hand and give me the key that would allow me to go on living without him. He'd tell me how to move on. He'd tell me not to be scared. He'd tell me what to do with the house, with Mummy, with Emma. He'd tell me how we could and would survive. But he simply couldn't write or direct that script.

I used to lie on his bed and stroke his hair.

'What's going to happen to me?' he'd ask, with the same petulance as a child asking how much longer before reaching the end of a long car journey. 'What's going to happen?' he'd persist, with the hospital mattress undulating beneath him, and the oxygen he hated so much whispering beside us.

'What do you mean?' I'd ask, volley-balling the question straight back to him. 'Can I do anything for you, Daddy? Anything? You mustn't worry.'

'No, darling. Nothing. Nothing at all,' he'd say.

And the moment had gone.

We'd talk about everything else, but not that. Not dying. He was able to say 'action' all his life, but now saying 'cut' somehow eluded him.

I'm not remotely superstitious. Never have been. I just don't believe in all that crap. I don't believe in signs or ghosts or that leaving one's hat on a bed is going to unleash evil spirits. I don't think a floating white feather is a dead person trying to make their presence felt. I don't even care about magpies; I'm always forgetting to salute them.

I used to think I didn't dream, and to be honest I was secretly glad. It meant I was incapable of boring people with those meandering, pointless non-stories over breakfast. But one of the unexpected side effects I blame on the chemo is how, every night, I hallucinate about newly hatched snakes. I think 'neonates' is the correct term for the baby ones. Mine are brightly coloured; yellow, purple and green. They aren't hurting me – they are just present. Sometimes I pick them up and play with them; wiggling them through my fingers like a reptilian cat's cradle. I'm not frightened.

I google what it means. Apparently, snakes evoke fear and respect. To dream about them means there is an enemy lurking. They represent a person who exhibits low, dirty, toxic or poisonous behaviour. However, they can also represent something that is related to health or healing. It sort of makes sense to me. I guess subconsciously I go to sleep fighting fear. I may not display toxic or poisonous behaviour, but the Red Devil is within me, seeping through my veins. I'm not scared in my sleep; I pick the little shits up and play with them. The Red Devil is my friend.

Health and healing. Healing and health. Sweet dreams.

There is a record I play on a loop whenever I'm in the kitchen. Katie Melua singing 'The Closest Thing to Crazy'. Not because I feel remotely crazy, but because right now I love and identify with two lines of the lyrics. They sing to me.

How can happiness feel so wrong?
How can misery feel so sweet?

Despite everything, I'm not depressed. I actually feel happy. Genuinely. I often find myself slipping the word 'gratitude' into a sentence. I used to always slightly mock the trend for being grateful for everything, from a cup of coffee to a sunrise, but now I get it. I'm grateful.

I feel more alive than I've ever felt, and I sort of love that feeling. An 'awakening'.

But there are other words I hate. I hate the word 'journey'. This illness is not a journey. Sorry, folks, but I don't regard going to the Cromwell for chemo, or lying exhausted on my bed watching afternoon TV, as a trip I'm remotely interested in taking.

Journeys always represent fun things to me. They are

getting up at 4 a.m. to board the Gatwick Express, trundling my suitcase down empty streets in order to catch an 8 a.m. EasyJet flight to Toulouse in the summer. That's a journey worth taking. Arriving at my friend Kathryn Ireland's farmhouse, year after year after year, trundling up the gravel drive in some shitty little car we've rented that has grinding gears and inefficient air con. It's honking the horn as we park outside the front door, every blue-shuttered window open wide, pink geraniums splattered like paint strokes in soil that's been dried out by the sun burning the earth. It's looking to the left and seeing a vast field of sunflowers standing tall. It's shouting to Kathryn, who appears at the window, leaning out, always in some sort of negligee, adjusting her voluminous breasts in welcome. It's the familiarity of arriving somewhere I truly love. Through the hall, into the kitchen, dumping my plastic bag full of British treats: *Country Life*, the *Daily Mail*, Cadbury's chocolate, Floris Lily of the Valley bath oil.

It's that first lunch in the cathedral-like barn with the fourth wall arched and open to the elements. Guests tumbling in, damp from the pool and freckled from having got a head start on the summer sun. It's the first snap of a freshly baked baguette and the first sip of chilled rosé. It's green beans and zucchini pasta from the garden drenched in home-made pesto.

It's lugging my suitcase across the drive to the converted pigeonnier and ripping off my London clothes and putting on a swimsuit, still smelling of last year's Ambre Solaire. The bed flat, with white sheets and thin eiderdowns, mosquito nets fluttering in the breeze. It's dumping my make-up bag in the bathroom and finding the shampoo I left behind last year still in the shower.

It's running through the spongy grass across to the pool, dodging the chickens and flopping on to a sunlounger. It's the music playing in the background and that hum of heat one only ever gets to hear in Europe. It's gossiping and laughing and tipping back bottles of Evian and opening a paperback and closing one's eyes against the glare of global warming. This is the *only* type of journey I'm ever interested in taking.

So whenever people refer to my cancer 'journey' I have a visceral reaction. I bristle. This is not a journey. This is a roller-coaster ride that I have no choice but to get on. I'm going to have to loop the loop, probably scream a bit, and do my best not to look down until the ride is over.

At the start of this ride, I had a very clear exit plan. My happy ending. I'd mapped it all out, with military precision. I imagined coming to the end of my six chemo sessions, getting rid of my gripper and port, and going straight from the second floor of the chemo ward to the Colbert restaurant in Sloane Square for lunch. Like a prisoner released from jail.

Real prisoners go through something called 're-socialisation', to prepare them for a new life in society after their release. After nearly six months of medically imposed isolation from everyone except my husband, I'll finally be physically reunited with my family. Out of solitary confinement. Resocialised. I'll be able to touch them for the first time in six months. I'll never let them go. Just thinking about that moment can make me sob in anticipation. Happy tears. I'll have both my grandsons in my arms. I'll hug everyone so tightly I'll probably give them the one symptom that originally alerted the doctors to my cancer in the first place. I'll make them breathless with my love.

I'll order chopped chicken salad studded with raw tomatoes (so not allowed on an alkaline diet) and overly salted French fries. I'll drink at lunchtime. A dirty martini. I'll gulp down the people I've missed so much. By then, surely, my sister and her family will be able to come home. Back to my home. There will be a Covid vaccine. Everyone will be safe. At present, that seems like such a faraway fantasy. The pot of gold at the end of the rainbow. But the dream keeps me strong and focused. I'm midway through being taught to meditate, and it's this scenario I replay in my mind as I learn to relax. My mantra isn't love or peace, or Krishna – it's family.

Family. Family. Family.

It's everything. More potent than any drug they can hit me with.

But alas, it's not going to be like that. Turns out I'll have to put up with delayed gratification. After chemo is over, I will be devoid of an immune system. My body will be totally spent. An empty vessel. Apparently, it takes a whole month to rebuild a broken body. Another month. Maybe longer.

Like Covid, cancer is the gift that just keeps on giving.

All my life I've been a sleeporexic. My childhood was spent either finding it impossible to go to sleep, or else waking up hours before anyone else. Or both.

My father was always sympathetic towards me. Being a night bird and an early riser himself, he was the one I would tiptoe towards when I had insomnia. Along the corridor, creeping down the stairs, past the cloakroom, into his study. The *clack, clack, clack* of his typewriter masking my silent entrance.

Daddy would be hunched over his messy desk, piled high with books, bits of paper and half-dealt-with mail, gardening brochures and random special offers torn from the back pages of the *Sunday Times Magazine*; half-smoked cigarette perilously balanced in an ashtray; whisky glowing in a chunky glass.

My childhood self glides to his side, and puts my little hand on his knee. He takes one hand off the typewriter and puts an arm around me. No words spoken.

'I just can't go to sleep,' I whisper, leaning my head against him.

'Do you want to get a book then, Flopsy?'

I nod.

It's our well-oiled, late-night routine. I nonchalantly

inch a piece of Juicy Fruit chewing gum off his desk without Daddy noticing, and walk over to the bookshelves. It's always a Nancy Drew girl detective I choose. I'm obsessed with this series of mystery books from America. They have titles like *The Secret of the Old Clock*, or *The Case of the Left-Handed Lady*, and I am a precociously good and avid reader. I devour these books, cracking their pale, yellow spines open and never growing tired of Nancy's plot-solving genius and her ability to suss out a crime.

I lie on the sofa, digging my feet beneath a cushion to keep cosy, and put the Juicy Fruit in my mouth. Every once in a while, I glance up at my dad, the back of his head haloed by the bright desk lamp. The clattering of the typewriter keys. The *z-z-zoom!* of the return. The pause while he lights another cigarette and rereads what he's written. This is my safe place from the night monsters beneath my bed.

Eventually, he finishes his writing, and we go through the cloakroom, up the stairs, along the corridor. He tucks me back into bed with my teddy bear and kisses my forehead.

'Go to sleep, Flopsy,' he says tenderly.

'One story,' I command. 'Just a quick one. A make-believe one.'

He lies down on my bed and starts a made-up story about a French cat called Monsieur Le Grand, who is outrageously naughty and lives off the rubbish put out by restaurants in Paris and has a gang of stray cats as his friends. I snuggle down and fall asleep, momentarily stirring as my dad turns off the light.

But now I face the endless nights alone. I sleep by myself, because I'm way too restlessly active to share my bed with Johnnie. Pre-cancer, I'd developed into a pretty lousy sleeper. I embraced the dawn. True dawn. It was quite normal for me to wake up at 4.30 a.m. and be awake for the rest of the day. I always woke up fully alert. Fully alive. When we shared a bed, I'd slither out and go into the kitchen and have my first cup of coffee. By 6 a.m. I'd be dressed and out to buy the newspapers from the corner shop.

Nowadays, I've taken my historic sleeporexia to another level. I do 'segmented sleep'. It's as though I'm a seventeenth-century farmer. Back in the day, segmented sleep was very popular. The nights were broken into two distinct sleeps, with an hour or two of 'quiet wakefulness' in the middle. This is now how I spend my nights. They seem endless.

My first, snake-dreaming sleep is a good, restorative sleep. I don't move. It ends at about midnight. From then on, it's party time. I'm fully awake. Alert. I switch on the telly, FaceTime my sister in America, drink hot water with lemon, and eat toast and Marmite. I read books, I potter about, I put face cream on.

At about 2 a.m., I put out the lights and try to force myself back to sleep. I'm hot, I'm cold, I'm turning the pillows, I'm panicking about everything. Life. Cancer. The future. Money. My port prevents me sleeping the way I want to sleep – on my stomach. I toss. I turn. I put on podcasts and hide my phone under a pillow so the light doesn't distract me. And eventually, restlessly, reluctantly, I succumb to another hour's sleep. If I'm lucky.

Nights are hellish. And I still wake up at dawn.

6

It's nearly Christmas. One day of the year; yet a day that carries great expectations. In my mind, it's become my fondly remembered record of family life. Mythical. The blueprint. It's all contained in that one day. To think back on Christmases past is like flicking through one of those Victorian moving-picture books. It's a measure of time. The history of family life, immortalised within a twenty-four-hour period. It's a day that's revered and looked back on with fondness – for me, and for all those blessed with happy childhoods.

My mother made Christmas the most magical time of the year – corny as that sounds. The build-up began with a trip to London to see Father Christmas at Harrods. Old Harrods. Good Harrods. Classy Harrods in its sixties' heyday.

When I was a child, Harrods was the closest thing England had on offer to rival Disneyland. Everything amazing and covetable seemed to exist there. From having my feet measured in a special X-ray machine twice a year for school shoes (whilst sitting like a princess in a swivelling circular chair) to buying party shoes. Party shoes were shiny. Sometimes red; more often black, with leather-covered buttons that required a special hook to do them up. I can remember parading up and down whilst my mother and the shoe assistant watched carefully, trying to detect any slipping of the heel. I was always impatient to get this bit of shopping over and done with, because I was completely indifferent towards clothes. And shoes. But my little sister wasn't. Emma lived for new shoes. She took forever choosing. She would sleep with them, still tissue-wrapped, beside her bed.

Emma was the extreme opposite to me. Ideally, I just wanted the convenience of dressing like a boy. I was at my happiest riding my bicycle, unencumbered by floaty dresses, and building highly complicated camps in the garden. Getting grubby. I used to make my body stiff and ugly whenever I had to try on dresses because I felt they were too constrictive. I was completely disinterested in their transformative powers. Emma rejoiced in being the pretty little girl she was. She loved twirling in front of mirrors, admiring her own reflection, and would have willingly sold her soul for any finery that was on offer. I was feral in comparison.

From Shoes we'd go up to Pets – a mini, indoor zoo. With the beauty of hindsight, this department was totally cruel and politically incorrect. It sold lion cubs, for God's sake. And massive snakes; their newly fed bellies pregnant with barely concealed live mice. We heard the noise of the animals before we entered the emporium itself. The excited barking of caged puppies, tumbling against the wire, throwing themselves at potential customers. The whiff of disinfected excrement. Reality snuffed out by sanitised consumerism. The kittens playing with balls of string suspended from the top of their cages; the lizards staring, unblinking, out of their glass boxes. It may be my fertile imagination playing tricks, but I think I remember once seeing a baby elephant for sale, cooped up in an open cage, its little trunk reaching out to passing customers. It was totally other-worldly. It was a pre-David Attenborough glimpse into the secret life of animals. As little children not yet infused with empathy, nor in possession of one iota of environmental conscience, I'm ashamed to say the only emotion these visits produced in me was a deep longing to buy. To have and to hold.

From there, it was up to the fourth floor. The Mecca. The toy department. The stuff of dreams. And Father Christmas himself. He was the real deal. None of this imposter shopping-mall shit our kids have to put up with nowadays. Harrods' Father Christmas came from the North Pole straight to the grotto. I waited in line, jiggling with anticipation. Head full of desire, whilst trying to remember to be polite and not just reel off my wants. Most of them came from the pages of a Littlewoods catalogue. A vast tome that Emma and I used to lust over in our nursery. Magic sets and sewing baskets. Jigsaws.

Bicycle horns. Board games like Risk and Careers. *Bunty* and *Beano* annuals. *The Guinness Book of Records.* Stiff little paper stockings with see-through netting on the outside, the middle stuffed with packets of Spangles, Jelly Tots, Fry's Five Centre bars of fruit-filled chocolates (gross) and slabs of Caramac. Tiny locked diaries with tiny little keys. We were lucky. We belonged to the generation devoid of electronics. Our imaginations not only fertile but boundless.

After Father Christmas, we would traipse around after our mother in the Food Hall. Our reward for being good was a box of Pierrot Gourmand lollipops to take home. Caramel flavoured. Not fruit. They were shaped like a large, inverted teardrop, and the trick was to put the whole thing in your mouth and suck and suck until you were left with just a tongue-ripping shard of see-through sweetness.

At home we always had a huge Christmas tree that reached up the spiral staircase in the hall. The lights broke from year to year, little bulbs painstakingly replaced, one by one, until they littered the floor. The fancy decorations unwrapped from tissue paper: the iridescent balls, the hanging icicles, the pre-tied, clip-on, perky red velvet ribbons, the wooden toy soldiers. All vying for branch space alongside the angels we'd made from loo rolls at school and the wobbly snowmen we'd constructed from stuck-together ping-pong balls.

I remember my mother circling the tree, making sure

it was decorated evenly. It was heaven. My father would remain totally uninvolved but would crank up the music in the drawing room, and I can still hear the echo of the choir from King's College, Cambridge. The evocative first solo chorus of 'Once in Royal David's City', gathering momentum as the rest of the choir joined in.

Our house was completely fabulous at Christmas. The fires were lit and crackling; black embers spitting and exploding under the fireguard like jumping jacks and occasionally burning little holes in the carpet. Christmas cards taking over the bookshelves. Big bowls of walnuts and pecans on the coffee table, with nutcrackers to split them in half. Satsumas with dried leaves still attached. So cosy and sweet smelling. It was close to paradise.

The endless, endless, endless wait before Christmas Eve. Being in bed a week before and suddenly hearing the tinny sound of carol singers coming up the drive. Running downstairs to watch them, forgetting to put on a dressing gown, the cold air hitting us as the front door was opened wide to reveal the majestic singing in the still night air. My father handing out port, then one final verse of 'We Wish You a Merry Christmas' belted out before Mummy pushed a folded one-pound note into the collection box, followed by tarnished, hot threepenny bits Emma and I had tipped out of our money boxes.

The kitchen and the larder were full. Getting food in for Christmas required major organisational skills in the sixties. Shops closed for days, and there were no cooking short cuts available back then. No prick-and-bake ready meals to fall back on. Everything was the real deal. We had to hoard. Plan ahead. So, Christmas cakes were baked and iced, puddings stirred with lashings of brandy added, hams cured and studded with cloves, a vast turkey delivered that sat in the pantry waiting to have those black, needle-like, stubbly remnants of feathers plucked. The milkman left pints and pints of milk, to see us through the holiday, and an entire wheel of cheddar.

We always got sent a hamper from Fortnum & Mason that was like a vast treasure trove of true exotica: Turtle soup, pickled walnuts, Piccalilli, china jars of anchovy paste, booze-infused marmalades, mustards, lemon curd, sugary glacé fruits. Emma and I would help dig out the contents; shaved ribbons of wooden packaging were sent flying across the floor. We personally found all the delicacies revolting, but we loved the concept. Basically, we just wanted the hamper to play in.

On Christmas morning, we'd wake up to bulging pillowcases at the bottom of our beds. Lumpy and enticing. Clock-watching until 6 a.m., before we'd drag the sacks of presents into our parents' bedroom, giddy with excitement.

'He's been! He's been!' Emma and I would scream, drunk with joy.

Our father would go downstairs to make coffee and I'd make a point of always eating a chocolate before I opened my first present. I still do. To this day, I can't start Christmas morning without a Quality Street.

Grandparents, aunts, uncles, cousins would all start to

arrive at midday; pillowcases now carefully stashed in our rooms, tissue paper trashing the floor of our parents' bedroom. We kids would be decked out in velvet dresses, our mouths full of crisps and sweets; the grown-ups much too busy to notice what we were doing. It was Christmas Day, and anything goes on Christmas Day.

The feast. The golden turkey, with everyone singing its platitudinous praise: 'It's lovely and moist, this year!' Virtually the only time of year the word 'moist' is vaguely acceptable to describe food – or anything else, for that matter. The stuffing, the gravy, the mountain of nicely burnt chipolatas, sprouts, carrots, red cabbage, roast potatoes and claggy bread sauce. I can still remember how it felt, looking down the big table, by now littered with torn crackers, unfunny jokes and useless trinkets, and thinking just how perfect everything was. How happy I was. How much I never wanted the magic of the day to end.

I still feel the same. The magic has never been diluted for me. Having children myself has only served to enhance my pleasure. Multiplied it. Sent it supersonic. And now having grandchildren, it's knocked the Christmas joy right out of the ballpark.

About five years before my dad died, the festive baton was passed on to me. I became the keeper of the flame. I'd still wake up at 5 a.m., heart pounding with excitement. The rest of the house fast asleep, I'd go into my kitchen, fiddle around with the last-minute food prep and crank up the cheesy Christmas music. I'd stuff my face with Quality Street whilst no one was watching, sort all the kids' presents into separate piles, and lay the crackers out on the table ready for lunch. The tree would be twinkling, black bin liners ready to collect the wrapping paper, candles lit and breakfast laid out.

But this year will be different. Fuck Covid. Fuck cancer. It will be a little Christmas. Just Johnnie and myself.

I can't even summon up the energy or impetus to get remotely excited about it. I'm no good at planning a festive feast for two. Fuck tradition, I'm going to go seriously off piste. I'm not cooking a turkey; that would be obscene. And ridiculous. It will have to be a minimalist Christmas. It will be like waking up in a sterile hotel room, when I prefer to be surrounded by clutter. A Tiny Tim of a celebration *à deux*; the children forced to create their own memories, away from me.

My mum is going to spend it with Elton, who is in her bubble. That thought snaps my heart into pieces. To be apart on Christmas Day. I can't actually think about it too much. The self-pitying tears come too readily.

I've bought a patio heater of great ugliness. It means I can see socially distanced friends outside my front door, without getting chilly. I've already started what I refer to as 'the withering'. I've rapidly lost weight; I feel the cold, having never done so before. I go to bed with three hot-water bottles. One for my feet, one for my back and one for my tummy. I sleep in sweatshirts. I shut the window. If I go out, I wear a woolly hat to keep the withering at bay. I'm dressed like Keira Knightley in *Love Actually* – except we've yet to get any snow.

Apart from feeling permanently chilly, I've escaped most of the hideous, more obvious side effects of the Red Devil, so far. No sickness, only a couple of mouth ulcers, no limbs swelling or tingling fingers. My temperature has been boringly normal. I fire what looks like a laser gun at my forehead six times a day. It operates on a traffic light system. Red – call the chemo team. Yellow – be careful. Green – pass Go, and live life with impunity.

Last night, Archie lent me Hank. Hank *does* have something wrong with his kidneys, as it turns out, but he's going to be okay. I got our next-door neighbour's daughter to walk him, as it was cold and pissing with rain, and whilst they were pounding the pavement I went to the loo.

Wiping my front bottom (as Nanny always euphemistically referred to it), my entire bush disappeared. *Whoosh.* Gone. No longer. I gave myself my first ever Hollywood. Painlessly. No waxing. No expense. Gone. In one go, I flushed it away.

I looked somewhat incredulously at my hairless minge, and then roared with laughter. The Red Devil must be doing its stuff. If it can give a sixty-one-year-old a porn star bush in one go, it's got to be doing its job.

It *must* be.

My hair is shedding. Fur balls litter my pillow. I call them fur balls. Other people call them angel wings. They have nothing to do with angels. They are fur balls.

They need the Dyson pet hoover to suck them up. There's nothing angelic about them. I've decided I'm going to do this in two stages. I'm going to have a short crop, before the shave. This devastates my mother. She belongs to that generation of women who manage to backcomb their hair and put on a bit of lippy in the recovery room after a hip operation. No joke. Their hair and keeping up appearances are everything to them.

'Don't cut it,' she advises, still convinced I am going to be the exception to the chemo rule. 'I'd wait.'

'For what?' I ask petulantly.

'Wait and see. You may be one of those people who don't lose much.'

'Mummy, I love your optimistic approach, but the oncologist told me categorically that with *this* particular chemo, and with *this* volume of chemo I'm having, it's a no-brainer. First thing I asked him.'

'Well, I just wouldn't.'

But I am. I've called my hairdresser. He's coming round on Tuesday.

The bush is just a taster for what's to come. I've crossed the Rubicon and there's no way back.

The withering has begun in earnest. Game on.

I was lying watching cartoons with Huck one Sunday morning, shortly after the first lockdown ended. We were playing a healthily competitive game of rock, paper, scissors. And he was getting bored with losing.

'Wait,' he said. 'I'm going to win this one.'

Back we go to playing.

I produce a fist: rock.

'I win, I win,' crows Huck, aged just six.

'I think you will find my rock beats whatever that is, you little weasel,' I say, tickling his bare tummy.

He's adamant. 'No, I win. Because I have the coronavirus on my hands, and the coronavirus beats everything. It can kill anything, it just goes *whoosh* into the air, and everybody dies.'

Fair point. Fuck Covid.

I don't like losing either. But I guess coronavirus is indisputably the Top Trump card to pull. Followed closely by chemo.

Unless you are Johnnie, who goes one further during our Annual Christmas Tree Row. He pulls the bloody cancer card.

I actually thought we could bypass the Row altogether this year, as one of the key triggers had been cunningly eliminated from the equation. This year, there was no buying of the tree in Battersea Park. The build-up to the Row – the selecting, buying and fixing to the roof of the car – wasn't there, because this year our tree arrived from Scotland. It was delivered. A thoughtful gift from Diana, who thought it might be nice not to have to bother with the usual routine. Not this year; what with me having cancer and being mid-chemo and isolating, and Johnnie complaining that he'd lost his core.

The Core – or, to be specific, Johnnie's Core – plays quite a starring role in this drama.

Johnnie likes to keep slender and fit, as he rightfully associates it with staying alive and being in good health. He walks daily, he tap dances, he moves. He's active. He does arm exercises and is forever working on his Core. He believes, at eighty-six, that his Core is not quite what it used to be, possibly due to the fact he had an eight-hour operation, aged seventy-four, for diverticulitis (which cut through every major stomach muscle he's ever owned), as well as having had a total of five hernias, one as recently as last year.

Anyway – back to the Core. The problem of the Core is one that Johnnie is constantly on a mission to rectify. It's all about reliable strength, as far as I can make out. He likes to be able to pick up heavy, inanimate objects like he did when he was twenty, and finds it frustrating when he can't. It's unacceptable. He also hates the fact he can't lay out wooden train tracks on the floor for Huck any more without needing the dual leverage of leaning on a sofa and a coffee table to get back on his feet. Understandable when you are eighty-six, I reckon. Totally excusable. Not to Johnnie. It drives him crazy.

He works on his Core when no one's watching. He does press-ups against tables and is adamant the Core is on the verge of a major Rocky-style comeback.

So, Christmas tree duly delivered the first week in December, courtesy of thoughtful Diana, we go about putting it up. It has arrived in a net condom, so it's very manageable.

'I've got a genius idea,' I volunteer. 'You get the tree

stand out of the hall cupboard, we plop it in, keeping the condom on, we tighten the screws, lift it up on to the table, and then – and *only* then – do we release it.'

This way, I reckon we won't be fighting with bits of stray branches poking one of us in the eye, which is what normally triggers the Annual Christmas Tree Row.

'Brilliant idea,' concurs Johnnie, already halfway up a very tall, unstable ladder in search of the metal tree stand.

I lift the tree up.

'What the hell do you think you are doing?' he screams from the top of the ladder, menacingly holding the heavy metal tree stand in one hand.

'Getting it ready to put in the stand. What do you think I'm doing?'

'Put it down, put it down!' he shouts.

'Stop shouting at me,' I reply, furiously.

'I'm not shouting at you,' he shouts back, coming down off the ladder and snatching the tree away from me. 'I'm doing this, not you. Sit down.'

I snatch it back, pine needles already shedding on to the wooden floor, dislodged by the violent tug of war that's taking place between the two of us.

'Give it to me,' I shout. 'It's heavy.'

'I know it's fucking heavy, you daft girl. That's why I don't want you to have anything to do with it. Go away. Leave it to me. This is one job I can do.'

'Your Core,' I say, full of spite and malice, striking a deliberate low blow.

Like Huck, he tries to Top Trump me.

'Your cancer,' he replies, triumphantly.

'My cancer?' I retort, grabbing back control of the tree. 'What possible difference does my fucking, spunking cancer make? Nice try.'

To prove my point, I hoist the tree up with one hand, plop it into the stand, screw the stabilisers tight and lift it, wobbling like crazy, up on to the table.

'See?' I say. 'I have both cancer *and* a core.'

We stare each other down.

'Fine,' says Johnnie. 'Have it your way, but the least I can do is cut the condom off.'

'Be my guest,' I say.

I walk over to Alexa and instruct her to play cheesy Christmas songs, *not* sung by Frank Sinatra, at volume 5. I know this will annoy him massively.

Johnnie takes a very sharp pair of scissors, perches on the back of the sofa, and proceeds to lean over the tree in an attempt to free it from its condom.

I say nothing. I just watch, hands on hips.

'Can I not help?' I goad him.

'No.'

Mariah Carey is going full pelt now in the background. 'All I Want For Christmas Is You'.

Tree finally freed and resplendent, I help Johnnie off the sofa and hand him a glass of wine, and we look at it. Together.

It's perfect. Perfect shape. The Annual Christmas Tree Row is over.

And cancer has triumphed over core.

7

It's 7th December and I've figured out something really important today. A revelation. I now acknowledge I must have felt like crap for about five months prior to my diagnosis. Cancer didn't just strike me out of the blue. I must have been so out of tune with my body that I failed to notice any telltale warning signs. I thought the dragging, full feeling in my groin was due to putting on 6lbs during lockdown. The fact that I'm middle-aged explained the need to continually get up in the middle of the night to pee. I imagined the weird itching of my thighs and buttocks was just an allergy; the strange welts that appeared out of nowhere were nothing to worry about. I even saw a dermatologist about it during one of the lockdown circuit breakers. He said it was stress. Or hives. A washing powder I was allergic to.

Wrong. Wrong. *Wrong*. Rooky error.

Today, despite having four ulcers in my mouth, rapidly thinning hair, and a porn star bush, I feel fantastic.

Really great. Better than I've felt in a long time. Last night, I slept for seven hours straight. I'm relaxed, I'm content. Happy with my lot.

I've come up with an analogy: if ever I have a car that goes wrong, starts smoking, makes a whining noise whenever I shift gears, or gets a flat tyre, I drive it to the nearest garage. I want to leave it with them to sort out. I hate it. And right now I feel that way about my body and my illness.

I'm going to hand this cancerous body over to the specialists, and I'm not interested in getting it back until it's perfect again. I'm not engaging in the broken version. Don't want the one that's got a port implanted beneath my breastbone, nor the one that's intent on producing fur balls, nor the one on a mission to wither. That body – that pathetic version of my body – needs to stay in the garage until it's fixed. Until it's been valet polished, has new brakes and is full of oil, gas and anti-freeze. Then, and only then, will I take back full ownership and drive off in it.

I can abide by this analogy I've come up with. I can relate to it. As long as I think of my body as a wreck that's been towed away to be fixed, I can do this. My sadness is that I can't rent a fancy new car to drive in the interim.

But after a good day, things turn ugly. Like a strange, sinister children's party entertainer who doesn't really care if the complexity of his tricks makes a child cry with frustration, my hair is now not performing well. Tonight, my mane has turned into a right royal diva. I'm shedding huge clusterfucks of fur balls every time I touch it. It's way too volatile and unstable to wash, brush or touch. I turn around and find I've left my mark: strands of hair lie at my feet on the kitchen floor. It reminds me of when India was sixteen and used to experiment with cheap, tacky, DIY hair extensions she'd buy in Brixton market. I'm not talking about a few stray tendrils, like when a baby grasps your hair and comes away with some strands; I'm talking about big chunks. And another one hits the floor. I am shedding.

I am talking on the phone, my mobile propped up by the sink on loudspeaker. Out of habit, I scratch my scalp. I come away with a big handful of hair. I'm incredulous. I stare at it because I can't quite believe this has happened to me. I get the hand mirror out and study the back of my head. I have a massive bird's nest of a knot. It's auditioning to become a dreadlock. It's as though Bob Marley's hair has mated with Amy Winehouse's beehive. I have a terrible feeling of doom. If I touch this wannabe dreadlock and try to untangle it, it's all going to fall out in my hand.

But this is the Red Devil doing exactly what it said it would do: it's taking away my hair. While it was still all there, I could sort of convince myself I didn't *really* have cancer. I didn't *look* like I had cancer. Now it's leaving me to face the music.

Only, my oncologist promised us more time together. It was one of the first questions I asked him. 'Will I lose my hair? How long have I got?'

He said it normally happens after the second session of chemo, and that's not for another week. Seven more days. That's what he said was normal. I've clung on to this time frame. This isn't part of the plan. This is too fast. I planned to have my hairdresser do a pixie cut tomorrow evening, but I think it's too late for that. If he combs it, I'm fearful it will all just follow my bush . . . and *whoosh!* Disappear. I don't know what to do. I am gripped by fear.

It reminds me of the first time I saw *Peter Pan* in the theatre as a young child. I was so traumatised by the thought of Tinker Bell dying, I shouted louder than anyone else in the audience. 'I believe in fairies,' I screamed. I was desperate to save that flickering light of hope. 'I BELIEVE IN FAIRIES.'

Problem is, this time I'm all grown-up and I don't believe in them. I can't save Tinker Bell, let alone save my hair.

But maybe AstraZeneca can save the world from this pandemic. The following morning, I wake up and watch the first person in the world being given the vaccine against Covid-19. I cry with happiness and hope. Ninety-one-year-old Margaret Keenan fearlessly takes one for the team. This is a historic day. It fills me with optimism and pride. If I were in charge of the government's PR team, I'd have followed her historic vaccination with one for Captain Sir Tom Moore.

I will always remember this day. There are certain

occasions in life that become microchipped into one's brain.

On 20th July 1969, my father woke me up, put a blanket around me, and he and my mum took me outside into the soupy night air. We stood on the damp lawn, and he made me look up at the clear night sky.

'Look at the moon,' he said. 'Remember this moment forever. This is history, you must never forget tonight as long as you live.'

We all held hands, the three of us turning our faces in unison towards the eternity of inky sky, stars and the shadowed moon above. It totally blew my mind. Neil Armstrong – an actual man, not a fictitious storybook hero – was walking on a planet zillions of miles away. Right now. In real time. I don't think I've ever felt as full of wonder as I did at that moment. Starry, starry night.

My dad had taken me to Virginia Water station, in 1965, to see Winston Churchill's coffin make its final journey from Waterloo to Hanborough. I was just six years old. The tiny station was packed with sombre, ordinary members of the public. You could hear a pin drop on the platform. A Union Jack flag was lowered in respect as the train crawled through the station. Hats were doffed, eyes lowered. It was a powerful, powerful silence. I stood stock-still, holding my breath, not fidgeting. Seeing grown-ups be sad was an alien concept for me. Haunting. The image will stay with me forever.

Johnnie and I have tried to do the same with our own children: these big, freeze-frame moments of life must be experienced so that they become seared into the memory. We took them to Kensington Palace to lay flowers when Princess Diana died. Tilly took her newly dead (and much loved) hamster, Jimmy Nail, tucked up in a festive biscuit tin lined with cotton wool. She loved him so much and had kept him in the freezer for a week. She wanted Diana to have his thawing corpse, as she'd read in a newspaper that she loved hamsters. No wilted flowers for the People's Princess from Tilly. No way. Instead, she got a semi-frozen and slightly putrid-smelling hamster. Respect.

I cry again when I see Matt Hancock get all emotional at the enormity of the vaccine breakthrough. I missed seeing him yesterday on television. I'm not the biggest fan of this government and their handling of the pandemic, but the pressure they have been under, and are still, must be monumental. Treading uncharted territory. Navigating a foreign landscape with no set of rules and no map. It must be like dancing in the dark; or trying to understand Braille if you're blessed with 20/20 vision. Impossible. Finally, though, it seems there might be a chink of light at the end of the tunnel. We may be on the brink of getting our lives back. One step closer to normality.

But I feel sorry for my sister and her family trapped in America, so far away from home. It *is* their home now, it's where they live, but I think home is probably far more potent than the country you live in. Home is always the place you want to return to when the shit really hits the fan. It's not where you end up. It's where you started in life. It's in your DNA.

And last night, my DNA meant that my hair gave in to the Red Devil. It capitulated. Waved the white flag of surrender. Exactly eighteen days after I started chemo, 99 per cent of my hair follicles went on strike. No gradual hair loss for me, what happened was more like Chernobyl.

I've called my hairdresser, Clive. I'm not quite ready yet for the fully shaved head. It's extraordinary how the mind clings to hope when you don't want to face up to something unspeakable. Like giving up smoking. You make deals with yourself. I remember when I finally gave up smoking for good, I used to yearn for just one more puff. It was an overwhelming desire; like wanting to sleep with an ex-lover after being cruelly jilted.

'If I just sleep with him one last time, it might not be really over. I might be able to get him back. I might be able to make him love me again. One more chance. Give me one more chance.'

One last cigarette. One more night together. A plea. I feel like that about my hair. Give us just one more week together. Seven days before I turn my back on you and walk away forever.

This evening, I open a bottle of red wine and pour Clive and myself a big glass. We are both cocooned in PPE.

Clive has cut my hair forever. He's dealt with the fallout of chemo many times in his career. He admits he's never encountered such speedy hair loss. He combs through the fur balls, and my hair just snaps. The cloud of weightless strands is the size of a football.

I don't sit in front of a mirror. Too brutal. 'Do whatever you can, Clive,' I tell him.

He sprays my scalp with water. He snips . . . and snips . . . and snips . . . and snips. I don't look down. Don't look at the floor. I sip my wine, lifting my double mask surreptitiously about a millimetre away from my face.

Snip. *Sip*. Snip. *Sip*.

I'm slightly drunk with sadness. I can't envisage myself with no mane. I was one of those fortunate babies born with a full head of hair and have basically never been parted from it.

My husband has stayed away. He's gone upstairs. He loves my hair even more than I do.

Snip. Snip.

Clive finishes. He looks at what he's achieved.

He sighs. 'I may have to come back next week and go shorter, darling.'

'Okay,' I say.

'And then when your wig arrives, I can cut that too.' He's trying his best to be non-emotional and practical.

'Okay,' I say. 'Just start a running tab and I'll pay you in one go.'

'I've cut your hair for thirty years. If you think for one split second I'm going to charge you for any of this, you must be crazy.'

Whoa. Kindness is so potent. It stops me in my tracks. I have to blink back my tears and stop myself from hugging him.

And I simply love my new haircut. As does Johnnie.

It is a fleeting love affair. Because two days later, I wake up to find I've got a bald patch. My parting is widening with alacrity. I pull a cashmere beanie on and wear it all day. Inside. In bed. In the bloody bath. I can't stand to look at myself.

I've sort of mastered this skill. I don't look at my port either, rising like a horrid, circular, lumpy doorbell beneath my skin. I get out of the bath, immediately put on a towelling dressing gown, and when I'm dry, I pull on a high vest. I don't think I'm vain. Well, no vainer than the next person. I think I just hate seeing myself as a 'cancer victim'. And I don't want pity. Nor do I want anyone to be nice and say any aspect of this actually suits me. Because they'd have to be lying. I wouldn't trust them. I don't want this particular badge of honour. And I think I might murder anyone who says I've got a 'great-shaped head'.

Surreptitiously, I text my friend Diana in the shop.

I need you to drop me off some vodka. Not a lot, because I might drink a lot if you do. A mini-bottle. I'm going to get Clive to come over and shave my head on Saturday night, and I can't ask my kids or Johnnie to do this. I need Dutch courage for this one. Or vodka. Probably both. Thanks.

I know she'll do it. No questions asked. She won't be

sympathetic and make me cry with her reply. She will be matter-of-fact. She replies immediately, in the middle of doing a £700 sale in our shop.

On its way. Sorry, but it's poncey stuff from Daylesford. The corner shop has closed since you've been sick and they always sold good battery acid.

That's my partner. Solid as a rock.

I don't know why I think my hair is such a fucking big deal. People lose limbs and man up about it. Logically, it is the least of my problems. I'm in lockdown. I can't see anyone outside of my house – or even inside my house, for that matter – for the next five months. I'm not trying to get laid. I have a husband who truly loves me. And yet. And yet . . . This is the one aspect of cancer that I thought, just like my mum, I might somehow be able to cheat. Deep down, I thought I might just prove to be an exception. But alas, as I keep reminding myself, I'm not that special. I wonder if my mum will finally believe me now? I wish I were special. But I'm not. I'm just a fucking bog-standard cancer patient going through savagely strong chemo.

Last night, I watched *First Dates* at 2 a.m. on catch-up when I couldn't sleep. There was a handsome thirty-five-year-old who was set up with a pretty thirty-something woman. They both made tiny talk. They sipped their cocktails awkwardly. They ate their scallops and their vegetarian mushroom starter. They got talking about their backgrounds and their families. The woman went first. And then it was the man's turn. He explained that he had been raised by a single mum he adored. And she got breast cancer when he was eighteen. And he said he didn't really take it on board at first. He and his brother were both typical boys and at an age when their selfishness was paramount. His mum was obviously his rock. His heroine. His everything. He came home one day to find she had no hair. Sitting at the kitchen table. Bald. And it destroyed him. He cried without shame, on prime-time TV. I felt his pain. And I knew, without a doubt, I don't want to put any of my children in a similar position.

I don't ever want my kids to have that memory of me. I want them to think of me always as their rock. I don't want to fuck up their lives any more than I already have done. I don't even want them to read this book until I'm back to being just their mum. Irritating Mum. Embarrassing Mum. Fun Mum. Healthy Mum. Normal Mum. It's massively important to me. Massively. It matters more than anything else. I want to be their fixer. I never want to be the person that needs to be fixed.

And I don't want anyone to take that away from me. That's my dignity gone if they do. Whoosh. Swish. Gone. Over.

So, shave on Saturday, hats for six days, and then a wig. A wig made from real hair. A bespoke wig that I've spent more money on than I dare own up to. A wig that comes from God knows where. Polish nuns? Nubile teenagers? Who knows? I've been measured, photographed, had cuttings taken of my hair before I lost it. I've been reassured that this is the real deal. A wig so expensive and fabulous no one will ever know the difference. I can blow dry it, cut it, curl it, shower in it.

But it doesn't arrive for a week. So, for a week I shall be bald, angry and bitter. And trust me, I will be all three.

But life marches on and this evening, wrapped up in a cashmere beanie, puffer coat, mask, gloves and scarf, I go to Warwick Square with Johnnie. We drive, because he is worried that I might get cold. It's 500 yards away from our house, yet he's right. I will get cold. I'm always cold. The Warwick Square Garden Committee is holding a carol service. A socially distanced carol service. So monumentally socially distanced, the thirty-five members of the choir are gated inside the two-acre garden. Sealed off with tiny little LED lights strapped to their foreheads so they can read the hymn sheets, and so their audience (pressed against the iron railings) can actually see them, because it is so dark. Not as dark as I am feeling tonight. I am murderous.

We meet my great friend Tricia, who is over here from the USA in order to direct two episodes of *Bridgerton* for Netflix. Her daughter and granddaughter are here too, and they meet us at the gates of the square. This is my big outing. The first in a month that doesn't involve a hospital. Yippee. I am pumped and have taken a large swig of Diana's vodka. I am also full of anger and self-pity and sadness, but no one can see that because it's dark and I'm double masked and am wearing my glasses. I am acting nice. Real nice.

And then the singing starts. And the choir's voices soar through the still night air. 'Once in Royal David's City'. 'Silent Night'. And then my fave. The one that always gets to me, even though I'm an atheist: 'In the Bleak Midwinter'. I have always got off on the funereal aspect of this carol. I love it.

I press my nose up against the railings, the spikey bits of holly just missing my cheek. I drink in the misery of it all. Johnnie leans up against me, and takes my hand in his. I know that he knows exactly what I am feeling. No words. That's the glory of marriage. There's nowhere to hide. Knowing. I wallow in the sad beauty of the moment. And I beg. I beg for Richard Curtis to do his magic. Please, Richard. Please. Because tonight, I'm crumbling. I'm not feeling brave tonight. Truthfully, I'm in despair. Help me.

And then it happens. I turn around and the tall, elegant houses of Warwick Square are all ablaze with light. The windows are flung open, the inhabitants are out on their balconies, their silhouettes shadowed, and clapping. Thank you, Richard. Thank you for this moment. You've done it. You've saved me. Truly. It is a sensational cinematic moment. You've made tonight okay. You've made me feel truly alive. Fuck it. Cancer, you're a cunt. You can take my hair. Have it all. Take it. No hair. Tonight, for a few magical minutes, I don't care.

My indifference is short-lived. Who am I kidding? I do care.

By the time I could walk, my mother was styling my hair into impressive topknots: not dissimilar to the kind

Yorkshire terriers are subjected to when they come back from the dog groomers. Only mine were lusher. Photographs from my childhood depict a round-faced little girl sporting fat bunches and glossy ponytails. Everyone in my family has got the gene. My mother, at eighty-seven, still has enviable hair, as do all three of my children. During my life, I've obviously ditched the topknots and bunches long ago; but never, ever the hair itself. I've never cut mine above my shoulders. Never been tempted to dye it blond, or auburn, nor succumbed to any fashion pundits advising women over a certain age to discard their flowing locks and adopt a more mature style.

I have loved my hair because it has never let me down. It has done as it was told, and we've never fallen out. Never fallen out until now.

When Johnnie has gone to bed, I sort of semi self-harm. I don't wait for Clive to come back and give me an even shorter pixie cut. No point. I brush my hair defiantly. Viciously. Multiple times. And every time, the brush has to be cleared of a huge fur ball. Into the bin it goes. By the time I've finished I look like an alien.

I look like someone who has cancer. And I feel unbearably sad.

I'm also sad because one of the best men on earth died four years ago today. Adrian Gill. I knew him for over twenty-five years and adored him. For a woman, there are few things as uniquely rare as a male friendship. It's like finding a pearl in an oyster riddled with salmonella.

And God knows, Adrian would have been the first to have ridiculed my analogy.

We both worked at *Tatler* together, before he was quickly poached by the *Sunday Times*. He was fabulously, wonderfully individual even then. He sported an affected and, I thought, totally pointless monocle, and wore heavy Sherlock Holmes coats (for no real reason other than the fact he liked the look of himself in them). Even then, Adrian didn't care what other people thought of him. He flirted. He teased. He was supremely certain of himself, and by golly he could make me laugh. And underneath all his certainty and self-confidence, he happened to be one of the kindest men I've ever known.

When he first separated from his wife and used to have his two tiny children, Flora and Ali, for the weekends, he would bring them over to me. Never with enough clothes, never sure how to change a nappy, never with a game plan, never remembering or finding where they'd left their shoes. We'd go off on adventures with my three children. Adrian could drive, but didn't want to, so we'd all pile into my pale-blue Toyota Previa, with Adrian sitting in the front seat, unapologetically chain smoking. The spirals of smoke infiltrating all five children's clothes. His bad language was exquisite. Beautiful.

It was during a period in my life when, every Saturday, Johnnie was performing in a West End matinee, and Adrian and I were like mismatched single parents. We'd gather up our kids and take them to parks, museums, a taxidermy shop on Westbourne Grove, bookshops, graveyards, restaurants – Alastair Little in Notting Hill, or Pucci Pizza in the King's Rd.

He'd invariably take my children to task about being 'provincial' in their food choices. He encouraged India to be adventurous by making her try oysters with mashed potatoes (her ordering) and teased Tilly about always wanting pasta and white food. He insisted everyone order ice cream for pudding, because he loved it so.

He managed to capture the children's attention because he could always answer literally any question they threw out. He never got bored with the annoying way small children keep asking insistently, only to drift off once you begin your reply. He had a knack of making everything interesting, and would add in a bit of anachronistic, superfluous information that would ensure they remembered his replies for the rest of their lives.

He taught me to make bitter marmalade in my kitchen and we'd spend a whole day boiling the Seville oranges, then slicing them wafer-thin, before adding the sugar and waiting while it bubbled and boiled into dark, unctuous, caramelised gunk. Adrian made delicious marmalade. One year, he didn't watch it attentively enough as it came to the 'rolling boil' stage, and it rolled and boiled into every crevice of my oven hob. And then he went home. He walked away from the carnage. I was incandescent. I used an entire box of Johnson's cotton buds trying to pick bits of orange peel out of the cracks and crevices. The next day, I received a huge bunch of flowers with no apology, just a note that said: *A big, sticky kiss.*

Adrian and then the love of his life, Nicola, and their two babes, were a big, rich part of all our lives. As a journalist, I would ring Adrian up and ask him if a sentence worked. I would go to his house for coffee, early in the morning when the twins were crawling round the kitchen floor, their little undone sleepsuits trailing behind them. We'd have supper. Lots of suppers. We'd go to the theatre. Celebrate Christmas Days together. India took care of their babies for nearly three years. It was her first proper full-time job. When my dad died, Adrian spent hours cooking an incredibly 'meaningful' dinner that contained both a boiled chicken and an egg – which had some ancient culinary and religious significance. Yes, he could be pithy, and pissy, and outrageously opinionated, but he was also one of the best men I've ever met. He was a multi-generational friend. A rarity. Across my entire family, everyone had an individual relationship with him, and adored him unconditionally.

Three weeks before he died, I'd asked him if there was anything he wanted me to do. He made me promise to always take care of Nicola and his kids, and asked me to cook supper at my house the following week, inviting six of our mutual friends and all of my kids. I cooked sausages and mashed potato, followed by ice cream. He liked all the food. I knew that this last supper was his way of saying an elegant farewell.

The day he died, I was in bed with tonsillitis. I think it was the first time as an adult I'd been totally felled by an illness. My throat was on fire. I had an earache like a five-year-old has an earache. Throbbing. A burning temperature. I knew time was running out for Adrian, but I still thought I had time to get better and to go and see him. To say goodbye.

India rang me. I could tell that she was driving but I couldn't understand what she was saying. She wasn't speaking, she was howling.

'Pull over. Stop driving,' I rasped.

'He's died, he's dead,' she sobbed.

I curled up into a ball on my bed.

Time stopped.

I will never not miss him. I probably would have shown Adrian my balding head. And he's not here to see it.

My baldness is getting ridiculous now. From Clive's cute pixie cut, I've gone to tufts in forty-eight hours. The parting is wide. I pull on a grey beanie and go to the hospital for bloods.

'Is there anyone here who could shave my head?' I ask nonchalantly.

'Let me see if Angela is busy,' says Lena, drawing yet another phial of blood from my arm.

I sit on a chair in the middle of the room, with a plastic apron made into a makeshift gown. I'm away from any mirror. I bow my head. It is the most massive act of submission I've ever undergone.

Angela buzzes the electric razor up the back of my neck. My hair falls to the ground. I see it out of the corner of my eye.

And again.

And again.

The bits by my ears.

I tip my head back, and she does the top, then gets a warm, wet flannel and cleans the stubble off.

'You've got a good-shaped head,' she says, standing back and admiring her work. 'Some people get buzzed and end up looking like an old walnut.'

I look at myself in the mirror, without seeing, and pull my hat back on.

I come home and keep my hat on.

I don't tell Johnnie what I've done.

I go into my bathroom and look at myself. After only one round of chemo, I'm a cancer victim. A goblin. I've got a walnut head. I'm both intrigued and appalled.

Hair goes with everything, and now I have none.

No floating up to the ceiling. No dissociating myself from what's happening to me this time, folks.

The mirror never lies.

8

What seems like the longest December in history crawls on. I spend my days going for mini-walks and cooking a bit and talking to friends and trying not to mind I'm not really a part of life as I knew it. I FaceTime both my grandsons, which I love doing. But it's not enough. It's not the same. I yearn to physically touch them. I see people on my doorstep, and then start to wither in the cold and have to stop. Once, I stood for too long gossiping with Nick and my godson Tommy, and genuinely thought I was going to faint. I stumbled backwards, clung on to a chair, and tried to pretend I was fine.

The withering is unstoppable now. My body is like an apple that got left on a windowsill behind a curtain. If I hold my arm out, the skin spontaneously ripples into that of an old person. Same with my thighs. Losing weight unintentionally is massively different than going on a diet. There's no pride in it; no sense of achievement. It's just scary. It makes me want to tell anyone who has ever complained about putting on a few pounds (and I include myself here) to simply stop. Stop worrying. Stop punishing yourself. It simply doesn't matter. When you are trying – and failing – to maintain your weight, you realise how pointless and frivolous trying to achieve a perfect body or an ideal weight is. Being healthy is all that counts, not being a perfect size 10.

Chemo makes nearly everything taste bad. Chemical. My mouth feels like I've licked a car engine. Only really strong flavours like Marmite cut through the grime, but even that is short-lived. Food offers no pleasure whatsoever any more. Tragic. I now eat to live, and that's joyless. For the first time in my life, I buy ready meals for the two of us. I prick-and-bake. I get excited when I see Marks & Spencer have brought out a range of Marmite-infused foods. Cream cheese. Butter. Crumpets. Pathetic, tiny, culinary nuggets that I can semi-taste.

Cancer is a relentlessly demanding mistress. It wants your dignity, your energy, your soul. Its prime mission is to suck the life out of you. Make you totally submissive to its every whim. It wants to control you.

I decide I'm not going to let it get away with this sort of behaviour. We are going to have a battle of wills. I'm prepared to meet it halfway, but I'm not going to put up with its petty tantrums.

One way I deal with this is to save nothing for 'best'. I tip double the number of drops of Floris Rose Geranium oil into my bath. I spray the hats covering my egg head with Fracas. On the days I bother to get dressed, I wear clothes I would normally 'keep' for special occasions. I use my nicest ribbons to wrap the scant Christmas presents I've managed to buy on Amazon. I read hardbacks in the bath, knowing the steam turns the glue in the spine sticky, and that if my dad were still alive, it would make him cross. I change my earrings often.

If I'm having a high-energy day, I exploit it. If I'm having a low-ebb day, I give in and go to bed. I feel no guilt. But I don't give cancer the oxygen it wants. I try not to let it bully me. I've become like my mother; fighting the ravages of age. Keeping up appearances. I wear make-up every day. I excessively moisturise and primp my skin. I can't backcomb like my mum does, alas, but I now understand the power of a bit of lippy and a smidgeon of blusher.

Nothing happens the second time I have chemo. Nothing. I have it and go home.

Like life in times of Covid, perhaps chemo will eventually become my new normal. Fingers crossed. Five days of steroids keep me busy, and I waited for the deep bone ache to attack, but it never does.

A welcome reprieve.

I hate the word 'fight' when connected to cancer. And 'battle'. Battle and fight both imply it's a raging war fought with a clear winner at the end. The reality is, it's not like that. It's putting too much pressure on the patient; the implication being if you don't get better, you're a loser. You should have tried harder. Everyone diagnosed with cancer tries their very best to get better. Trust me. Everyone is a fighter. Everyone's a warrior.

I try to use another word. Thwart. 'I'm trying to thwart cancer.' To thwart is to attempt to foil.

It's impossible for anyone cancer-free to understand just how hard you try every second of the day to keep going. You try to remain upbeat. Positive. Cheerful. Grateful. It's impossible to leave out grateful – you're urged to feel it constantly. You put up with indignities. Loss of freedom. You throw away your old life. Your old looks. Your vanity. You try to choke down food that you can't taste, wear clothes that no longer fit, look at a face you struggle to recognise. You hand over your body to science. You relinquish control. You try not to project your fears on to the people who love you the most. You give it your best 24/7.

When you are the one who has cancer, it's hard to live in anything but the moment. Day by day. You start out with a clear plan, laid out by doctors and oncologists – in my case, six rounds of chemo in three-weekly cycles – but it's naive to assume that this schedule is set in stone. Shit goes down and you have no choice but to roll with the punches. Crack on and try to keep calm.

I liken it to having an infestation of mice in the kitchen. You see one hugging the skirting board, so you buy a trap. Nothing happens, except that the cheese you've set in the trap dehydrates. You up the ante and lay down the carpet of death – or as we euphemistically call it in our house, 'the stairway to heaven' – those uber-sticky tiles that mice are supposed to never be able to escape from. And you wake up one morning and find a minute character from Beatrix Potter jerking about as though electrocuted, and you feel utterly wretched. You feel dreadful until you see its little friend, Hunca Munca, scuttling about the following night and you decide to call in Rentokil. The hit men. You want those little buggers out of your kitchen. Forever. Humanely, inhumanely, you don't care. You just want them gone. I feel the same way about cancer. You start out thinking the cure is going to be linear, simple. Humane even. You quickly realise that it never is.

Before I got cancer myself, I read fairy tales about people who managed to get rid of hideous diseases through juicing and crystals and meditating. Flying to Mexico for exotic cures. Maybe the tales are true, but I'm a realist. I have zero faith in ineffectual traps and sticky paper. I don't think they work. I want the medical equivalent of Rentokil to come in and mass-exterminate every raddled cell in my body. I choose to believe in the science.

And then I get thrown my first truly terrifying cancer curve ball.

Having plundered Amazon Prime for necessary home medical monitoring equipment (an oxygen reader, an electronic thermometer, a blood pressure and heart rate machine), I take my own readings. Daily. Sometimes twice a day. My heart rate – normally coming in at 85 beats per minute – has gone crazy. It is 215. I can feel it. I can see it. My heart is fluttering beneath my nightdress.

Staying calm, I replace the batteries in the machine and have breakfast before trying for another result. 220. I feel dizzy, spacey. Scared. Really thrown.

I ring the hospital oncology ward who say to come in immediately. And if I am too far away, to call an ambulance. Johnnie drives me there. Fast. Though nothing is speeding as fast as my heart. It is going at full throttle. I have the window open to try to steady myself, but my heart is breaking. Literally. I can feel it breaking free from my chest. It is terrifying. My poor Johnnie has to drop me off at the front door; Covid allows for no hand-holding or visitors. He is bricking it. As am I.

Up to oncology ward where they are waiting for me. I am spread out on a reclining chair. One nurse takes blood from my right arm, one from my left, whilst a third nurse reopens and flushes out my port so that they can collect blood straight from there. They wire me up to an ECG machine and take my blood pressure.

Boom. Boom. Boom.

My heart is now kick-boxing inside me.

I can tell by the volume of bloods taken, and the speed at which the nurses are instructing it to be tested, this is no joke. The constant fear during chemo is sepsis, which apparently can happen very fast, as the immune system is so compromised.

I'm sent off in a wheelchair for an echo cardiogram. But my heart is beating so quickly they have to abort the test.

Boom. Boom. Boom.

Don't go breaking my heart. Please. I beg you.

Now I'm moved to the cardiology ward. Nurses come into the room constantly. I call Johnnie and I can hear his voice tighten with fear. Mine is just a whisper.

I see three different cardiologists. One makes me try an exercise which sometimes manages to get the heart out of this rhythm. For this is what has happened. I'm not having a heart attack. Although it sure feels like it. My heart has short circuited, or created a new circuit, and needs to be jolted back into its old pattern. To stop doing the tango and go back into doing a slow waltz. The exercise relies on the same method of bearing down and breathing I remember being taught during childbirth classes. I'm quite good at it. I can keep bearing down and going puce in the face and not breathing for a very long time. I've remembered how to do it after all these years. Hell, I'd have pushed this phantom baby out easily. But my heart remains disco dancing inside me. 215 beats. Then 218. Back down to 215. Back up. Now 221.

Another specialist comes in and says he wants to try performing a deep massage on the vein in my neck. He does quite a painful manoeuvre, which feels not dissimilar to slowly being strangled. My heart is defiantly pounding away, totally resisting any attempt to get it to pipe down.

Now things really get moving. Nurses come in and start snapping on blue gloves. They line up against the wall opposite me, looking like masked cast members of *ER*. A student nurse joins the party. Then my oncologist appears. Two cardiologists. It's crowded. I'm panicking.

'Okay, Sarah, what we've decided to do is we are going to give you something that stops your heart for about ten seconds. It feels a bit strange, and I can't pretend people like having this done. But first you will feel a heaviness on your chest, and then heat.'

I love the way medics never give you an option. *We are going to give you something that stops your heart for ten seconds.* Think about that sentence. Or better still, don't. That's quite a punchy showstopper, and yet it's delivered with the same casual intonation as announcing 'dinner is about to be served'.

Ten seconds. Heart stopped. One. Two. Three. Four. Five. Six. Seven. Eight. Nine. Ten. Count it out. I dare you. It's longer than you think.

I strangely know what it is they're about to do to me. Three months ago (when I actually enjoyed and relished watching life-and-death hospital documentaries on TV), before I had cancer, I saw this done. It was on an episode of *24 Hours in A&E*. And I've remembered it. There was a sixteen-year-old boy who'd been rushed into hospital with terrifying heart palpitations and was in there with his dad. It had obviously happened to this kid before, because the documentary showed him pleading with both his dad and the doctors not to do it. It made me nervous.

I have been given no choice.

'Okay, but you have to promise to talk to me while you're doing it,' I say. 'Promise me that. Throughout. No silences.' Part of me is petrified, and part of me is morbidly fascinated. Dying for even ten seconds – because surely that is what having no heartbeat must feel like? – might be like a dress rehearsal. I might come out the other side having had a sneak preview of what it feels like to no longer exist.

I am given a slow injection. The doctor talks. They've promised me they'll talk to me, and they keep that promise.

'Right. We're going in now. You are going to feel a weight on your chest. And the heat spreading . . .'

Yes. Yes. Yes. Help me, God. I feel weight on my chest. I feel that. I'm looking straight ahead at the sea of medical faces and now I'm waiting. I'm waiting for . . . what? What am I waiting for? A white light? My whole life to flash before me? To die? I don't know, but nothing happens that I am aware of. I'm guessing my heart stops and is rebooted. Because here I am. Alive. It is all a bit of an anti-climax.

'Well done. You did brilliantly.'

It's over. It's done. I'm rebooted. I've briefly flatlined, but I'm back in the game. My heart is slow waltzing like a geriatric at a cruise ship's tea dance. But after one hour, it misbehaves again. It stops waltzing and goes into a samba.

I'm made to go through the same procedure again.

And once more, only with twice the dose of medication.

By now I'm an old hand. Stop. Start. Stop. Start.

Second time, I'm lucky. Third time, I'm still alive.

The rhythm stays put. My heart belongs to me again. I'm unaware of its presence for the first time in eight hours.

I didn't like feeling bionic. It was the only time during this whole medical cancer diagnosis I thought I might die. But I didn't.

I'm here. Still standing.

9

When India was just six weeks old, we moved to America. Johnnie was playing the lead in a huge American television series with Robert Wagner, and Westwood, California was to be our new home. We'd been married for just over a year, and life had never been sweeter. I was twenty-five and Johnnie forty-nine. He was an established and highly esteemed theatre actor, at the peak of his career in England, and I was a precocious published author with a book of tortured poems beneath my belt as well as a series of articles in *Ritz Magazine*.

Starring in an American television series was like winning the financial jackpot for a working British thesp. No more rehearsal rooms in Acton, no more glory jobs for minimal wages working at the National Theatre, no more Wednesday and Saturday matinees, no more dog-eared scripts with cues highlighted in marker pen, no more mornings with me spent listening to lines, no more nightly nerves kicking in at 3 p.m. or me waiting up until

10 p.m. in order to jump on the bus to meet him at Langan's Brasserie for a post-theatre dinner.

'We are going to be officially nouveau riche,' declared Johnnie excitedly when the deal from ABC was finalised. 'And guess what? I'm being given my very own Winnebago.'

A Winnebago. Can you even imagine what being given your own Winnebago is like? We couldn't. We simply couldn't believe our good fortune.

We were in Venice, staying at the opulent Danieli Hotel, when the call came through from his agent. Sitting up in bed, drinking fresh orange juice and dunking crumbly pastries festooned with little white pellets of hard sugar into bitter coffee. I was about three months pregnant. It was the first time I'd ever been to Venice and everything about it was magical. It was snowing and the lagoon was semi-frozen. The vaporetto had to snap through thin shards of ice to reach our hotel, and the mist totally enveloped us. When the outline of the magnificent buildings rose hazily before us, like some giant wedding cake, appearing as if by magic, I cried with wonder. Uncontrollably sobbed.

The romantic in me – then, and on every subsequent visit – always imagines what it would be like to be deeply unhappy in Venice. I fantasise that I have an internal soundtrack of the most heartbreaking opera arias accompanying me across the cobbled squares, the music swirling around the marble pillars. I visualise what it might be like to sit in Florian's alone, sipping a hot chocolate; watching my tears in the distorted reflection from the green-patinated mirrors. What does this say about me? In my life, I hate unhappiness. And I avoid it whenever I can. Venice is the most haunting backdrop to misery and abject loneliness; yet I've only ever known supreme happiness and good times there. Go figure.

We flew to America and bought a house. A picture-perfect, clapboard 1920s home with wooden floors, four bedrooms, and a little enclosed yard with lemon trees and cobalt-blue agapanthus. It still had all the original tiles in the bathrooms. The kitchen boasted the original oven, with kitsch built-in salt and pepper shakers, and a griddle to make waffles. There were remnants of what must once have been considered 'mod cons' – an ironing board, hidden in a long cupboard, that fell into place when you opened it, a thinly disguised safe under the staircase, and a spice cupboard. We loved it for all these quirks and kept them, like objects from a bygone age that linked us back to England. Americans' appreciation of old when it comes to houses is different than ours. They don't really cherish old. To them, we had bought a 'tear-down' – to us, we had bought character and charm. We were enchanted.

We were paid a 'relocation moving fee' and we spent a lot of it on a beautiful Biedermeier table and lily of the valley fabric from Colefax and Fowler to use as curtains in our bedroom. We rented out our house in Fulham, and shipped a lot of our belongings over to the States. A team of Mormon builders knocked down some walls, repainted others, and installed a highly sophisticated alarm system. Gardeners replanted the garden with exotic indigenous plants and built us a wooden deck.

Robert Wagner's assistant oversaw the renovations, because Johnnie was still working in London, doing a Tom Stoppard play at the National. Three weeks after India was born, he flew off to Amsterdam to film the first episode of the American series, entitled *Lime Street*, and the plan was that I should fly out to Los Angeles with our baby, taking our doctor's twenty-one-year-old daughter, Sophie, with me to lend a helping hand.

We stayed at Robert Wagner's ranch in Brentwood so that I could furnish the house, ready for Johnnie's arrival. In retrospect, I had zero notion what I was doing. I was a child. A complete novice. I would swan into Bullock's, the local department store, with India strapped to my chest and wander around the homewares department, recklessly gathering up oversized towels and brightly coloured Fiesta Mexican plates. I bought beds and washing machines, and unpacked our shipped belongings. I played at Mummies and Daddies, with my oversized Wendy house and my little live dolly. I wanted it to be a real home for Johnnie when he got back. I wanted to be the perfect housewife.

There was only one problem. I couldn't drive. To live in Los Angeles and not be able to drive is akin to being a leper. Luckily for me, Sophie drove – but obviously this wasn't going to be a long-term solution.

'As soon as you pass your driving test, darling, I'd

love to buy you a car of your choice,' said my newly nouveau-riche husband one night, calling all the way from Amsterdam.

'Seriously?' I said.

'Nothing would give me greater pleasure,' he replied.

I put down the phone, snapped India into her car seat and made Sophie take me to the driving test centre on Pico Boulevard in our rental car. First, I had to complete a written multiple-choice quiz. Tick the boxes. Questions like 'If a child ran into the path of your car would you: a) accelerate, b) swerve, or c) brake?' I passed.

Next up: the practical bit. A Mexican instructor got into the car beside me. The car was an automatic. I drove around the block three times, using my indicator and checking my mirror, I stopped at the stop sign, drove back off, pulled out from the pavement, and parallel parked. The instructor loved my English accent. He was impressed. Seduced. I was now the proud owner of a Californian driving licence.

Next up: the car. We drove straight to a dealership. I wasn't fussy. Ford was the first one I saw, the only one I was aware of, and I immediately fell in love with a cream-coloured Ford Bronco. The same truck O. J. Simpson would flee in, pursued by the police, when he was facing arrest in 1994. I knew sweet nothing about cars. Or trucks. But I knew this one had my name written all over it. It was high off the ground, with a big trunk, and it had a CD player. I bought it with my pristine, newly acquired American Express card, and drove off with the ink not yet dry on my temporary driving licence. I strapped India into her little bucket car seat, cranked up the radio, opened the window and headed home. Freedom.

If Johnnie was surprised to be met by me at the airport, three days later, he didn't show it. Nor did he appear amazed that his wife had chosen an unlikely and distinctly unglamorous vehicle in which to get about Hollywood. However, no amount of acting could disguise his sheer terror when I got behind the wheel and started actually driving him home. With our new baby.

He white-knuckled it for about five minutes, then made me pull over. At that stage, I'd probably got a maximum of six hours' driving experience under my belt.

'I'm going to take over,' he calmly announced. 'You sit beside Indie in the back, in case she wakes up and needs feeding. I'll drive us home.'

Now Johnnie was back filming in America, his schedule was gruelling. He'd leave for the studio at dawn and return after I'd put our baby to bed. Every evening, pink pages of rewrites would be delivered. New lines to learn for the next day. Sometimes I'd meet him for lunch in his Winnebago, which had been kitted out to cater for his every whim. The fridge was filled with apple juice and Diet Coke, huge bowls of oversized fruit sat on the counter, and tall vases were stuffed with constantly renewed displays of flowers. He had his own 'hunker' – a man just waiting to fulfil his every need. Not only were we nouveau riche, Johnnie was treated like a potential diva.

Meanwhile, back at our home, I would receive eggshell-blue Tiffany boxes from people I didn't know, containing silver photo frames engraved with our child's name. 'Welcome to LA', the gift card would read. Giant teddy bears with satin bows would be delivered from faceless executives at the TV network, gingham-lined baskets of cookies and muffins, invitations to parties from people we'd never met. We were the new kids in town. Fresh blood. And we were British. And I was so lonely.

I was set up on a blind date with a woman whose daughter was the same age as mine. A friend had sat next to her on a flight from London to Los Angeles. By some karmic twist of fate, they'd discovered they both had god-daughters the same age, and they decided to put us in touch with each other.

So I decided to cold-call Tricia Brock and invited her to our house to have lunch with her baby, Cleo. Tricia was from Missouri and was a script writer. She accepted the invitation, and I went all out. Overachieved. I laid the table with a brand-new tablecloth and napkins, bought supermarket flowers, and decided to make a spinach soufflé. My speciality. Tricia was in her early thirties, and I wanted to impress her with my sophisti-cated housekeeping. She was late, but I managed to hold it together, salvage the soufflé. Despite the fact it was about 99 degrees outside, we placed our two sweaty babies side by side on a blanket next to us and awkwardly got to know each other.

Like all new mothers, the conversation quickly turned to Top Trump childbirth stories. Hers was natural, long, painful and traumatic. Mine was embarrassingly easy: epidural, short and sweet. We were like Jack Sprat and his wife.

'Do you think you will ever have sex again as long as you live?' asked Tricia in her fabulously sexy accent.

'Well, actually, I'm six weeks pregnant,' I confessed, caressing my stomach.

Tricia pushed her chair back from the table, lay on the floor with her legs in the air, and howled with laughter and disbelief.

'You have to be joking me,' she roared, clutching her vintage floral skirt with one hand and adjusting her sodden breast pads with the other.

'Nope,' I replied. 'I am.' I went and lay beside her, next to our babies.

That was the start.

We've been best friends for thirty-five years. As have our daughters.

Fast-forward three and a half decades.

Tricia and I are both grandmothers, sharing that unique passion for our children's children that I liken to being injected with love heroin. Oceans normally separate us, but our friendship has remained constant. We share the history of our youth. And as we get older, that familiarity becomes even more precious.

Just as I get diagnosed with cancer, Tricia's daughter

moves to London. And not long afterwards, Tricia lands a massive directorial job for Netflix, which is to be filmed here. We're together again. Close.

Most days, Tricia walks from her hotel, no matter what the weather, and stands on my doorstep. I can't retain heat, so I stand, bundled up in hats, scarves, gloves and padded coats, with my ugly patio heater dragged on to what she calls my 'stoop'. We talk. Seeing her in person is the most wonderful, unexpected gift. Sometimes she brings her edible, Polly Pocket-sized granddaughter Tallulah with her. Watching them together is like rolling back the years to when we first became friends.

Two days after my second dose of chemo and the terrifying stop-start heart incident, Tricia tells me she's going to drop by in the early evening to say goodbye. She's heading back to New York to pack up her apartment before returning, after Christmas, to start filming *Bridgerton* at a studio near Heathrow.

It's ten days before Christmas. I feel I've crammed so much drama into the days already that to actually survive long enough to reach the main event will be nothing short of a miracle. Although I pretend to all and sundry that I don't mind the fact that Christmas is going to be very different this year – for everyone – I do. I care. Desperately. I'm totally gutted. I'm gutted we're all in lockdown again. I'm gutted I don't get to see my family. I'm gutted I've been forced to buy sub-standard presents on the internet. I'm devastated that I've needed to farm out my children's embroidered felt stockings to their

individual homes, instead of creating the usual festive clusterfuck across our mantelpiece. I'm devastated
that I haven't even bothered to get out the vintage
painted blocks, unwrapped year after year, that spell
out 'M-E-R-R-Y C-H-R-I-S-T-M-A-S' across our windowsill. Nor have I decorated our tree with anything other
than basic coloured lights. I just don't have the energy.

Christmas is normally the highlight of my year. I love
the cooking, the smells, the family traditions. It's more
than just a day to me. It marks the passage of time, like a
secret one can revisit to recall the highlights of family
life.

There was the year after India and Sean got married, when they went to Mustique for Christmas. It was
also the first Christmas my dad was no longer here, and
I had my first drink at 10.30 a.m. to numb the pain I
felt. We were altering the ground rules, in an effort to
pretend we were all coping; moving out of our comfort
zone. We weren't celebrating at our home; we were
going to my friend's house instead. Changing the venue.
We got a FaceTime call from India, just as I was being
spat on by the chipolatas I was cooking on tinfoil to
take over to Phoebe and Charles's later. Tilly picked up
the call.

'Happy Christmas, darlings!' I shouted from the other
side of the kitchen, my head buried in the oven, my hot
tears hidden as they plopped on to the baking tray. I
didn't want to ruin their day by letting any of them see
I was upset. But I *was* upset. I missed my father, and

I hated seeing my mother put on the bravest of brave faces, and I hated the fact I was without one of my children for the first time ever.

'Go get Dad,' instructed India. 'Where's Archie? Get him too. I want to wish you all a Happy Christmas together.'

I dashed away my tears and shouted for Johnnie and Archie. I had a little crack in my voice.

India and Sean were standing in a brightly lit, tiled bathroom. Sun-kissed and loved-up. India was in a bikini and Sean had one arm draped around her.

'We just wanted to tell you what your Christmas present is from us,' said Sean, once we were all gathered round the laptop. He paused, pulling Indie towards him. They were both grinning. 'Happy Christmas, Granny and Grandpa.'

Time stood still. My life went from black and white to Technicolor. The plot twist, and their happy news, transformed a melancholy day of false bravado and sadness into a crescendo of endorphins, pregnant with hope for the future. What ultimately turned out to be Huck was sitting inside India's belly, like a much-needed Band-Aid of love. A little nugget of happiness. A promise. He mended us, that year. And back then, I naively imagined that sad Christmases were a thing of the past.

But 2020 has been a bastard of a year. Christmas promises to be a cancerous, Covid- and chemo-ridden brute. A reduced holiday. Pared down and diminished; with families forced into bubbles and given strict instructions as to how they can enjoy their celebrations. Matriarchs across the country are deemed too old and vulnerable to be with their kids and grandchildren, for fear of catching the virus; grown-up children are faced with the Herculean task of cooking Christmas lunch themselves for the first time ever. No big gatherings, just pods of people trying to juggle which members of their family they can justify having round their table without breaking any lockdown rules. It is joyless.

Johnnie and I are obviously going to be alone this year. That is a given. No mess, no festive feast, no chaos. It doesn't feel like a celebration to me. There is precious little to celebrate, let alone with any oomph. So why bother? The one year I would have loved, more than anything, to have all my family under one roof, it is deemed impossible. It is a case of fuck Covid, fuck this cancer of a cracker. Bah humbug – with bells on.

The doorbell rings.

'That will be Tricia, come to say goodbye,' I yell at Johnnie.

I grab my coat and gloves and open the door. It has just rained and the moisture sparkles, caught by the street lamps, throwing shards of light like razors across the pavement.

Tricia is standing in front of me with her daughter Cleo holding little Tallulah's hand, but I am confused. The street is filled with people. They are all wearing scarlet cloaks and holding lanterns. There is music coming from a CD player to my left. My first thought is that, for the first time ever, our 'hood has been invaded by carol singers. Improbable. But possibly possible.

'We Three Kings of Orient Are' rings out beside me, cutting through the silence like a sword. I look across the street and see a hooded couple standing with their arms around each other. And then, out of nowhere, Archie's dog runs into the house. I am utterly disorientated at the sight of Hank. I look back at Tricia, and then, to my right, I make out Archie holding little Billy in his arms, stiff as a poker in his snowsuit and wide-eyed with wonder at being out in the dark. And there is Nisha beside him. Grinning. A cluster of people cross the road, and suddenly I see Huck holding India's hand, and I burst into tears. These aren't just random carol singers ringing my doorbell; these are my family and friends. There is Anya and her husband James with their children, huddled next to Tilly and Felix, India and Sean. They are all here. I can't touch them, but I am being given the tightest embrace I've ever felt.

It is Christmas, past, present and future, all rolled into one; like a Pass the Parcel of love. Each carol, each layer, slowly unwrapping before me: 'Silent Night', 'Hark! The Herald Angels Sing'. These are all my angels, standing before me. I just drink in the total perfection of the night. I am overwhelmed by the thoughtfulness and kindness. Tricia has organised a surprise party that surpasses all surprise parties. This is my Christmas. Socially distanced but squeezing my heart to bursting point.

My eyes circle the horseshoe of people, seeking to freeze the frame of happiness I feel. Preserving it. Forever.

I wake up on Christmas Day itself and feel devoid of the normal adrenaline rush of urgency. I go upstairs and try to get it back. To pretend. To dupe myself. I eat two Quality Street before breakfast – the orange cream, followed by the flat toffee – and switch on my Christmas tree lights. No turkey to baste, no sprouts to peel. No grown-up children asleep in their childhood rooms, no chance of making so much noise I might succeed in waking Huck and whipping him up into a fever of excitement over the fact that Father Christmas has come. No row of embroidered stockings hanging, plump and enticing, on the mantelpiece. That makes me feel sad. It is the first time in thirty-five years I haven't been able to fill my kids' stockings.

Even without Boris Johnson's hastily issued instructions that this Christmas needs to be shrivelled and shrunk into a pick-without-the-mix December 25th, mine was always destined to be a mirage of normality. Our house with its half-hearted decorations, mere props, carries a tangible atmosphere of Groundhog Day. I make a cup of coffee, and text India.

Please, please, please will you FaceTime me when Huck wakes up so I can see him opening his stocking?

Even as I press send, I know this will be an annoying request. I am asking them to be distracted from their first-hand pleasure by a screen, and to blurrily convey

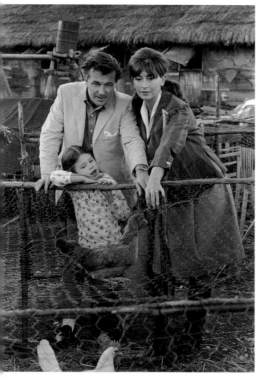

Visiting my parents on the set of *King Rat* –
loving the chickens. Los Angeles, 1965.

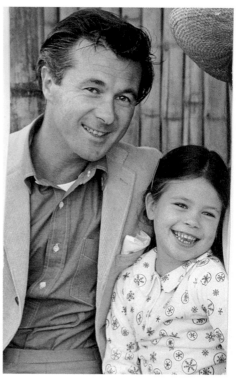

Me and my dad.

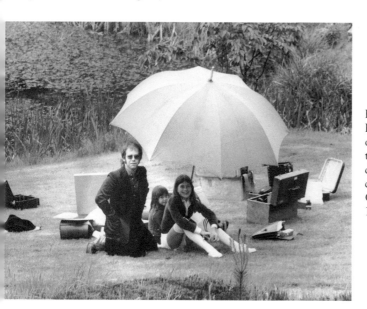

Elton John, my sister,
Emma, and me in
our garden during
the filming of a
documentary that my
dad directed, called
Goodbye Norma Jean.
1976.

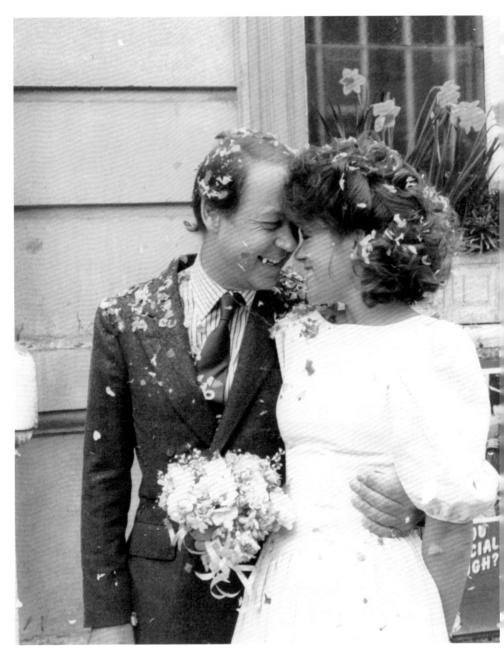

Big hair for my wedding, 1984.

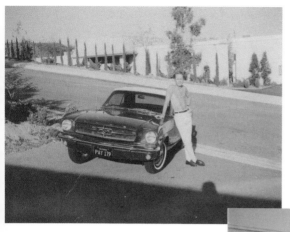

Johnnie showing off both his Mustang and his core. Los Angeles, 1965.

Me, aged 5. The way we were when we first met.

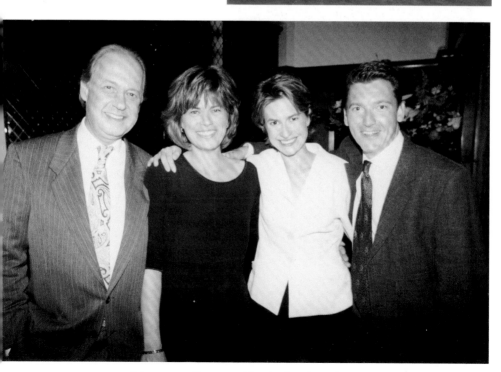

Johnnie, me, Emma and her husband, Graham.

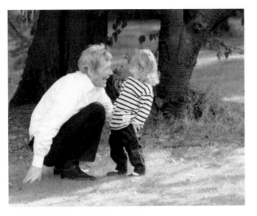

My daughter, India, and Peter O'Toole.

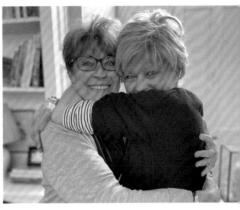

Me and my mum.

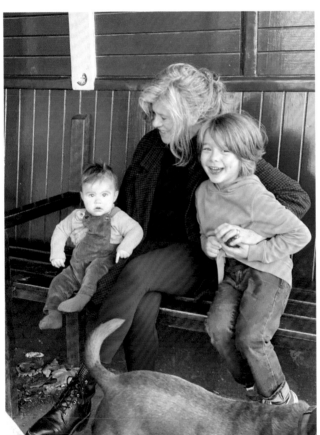

This photograph makes me both happy and sad. I had just been diagnosed with cancer, and was starting treatment the following week. I still had hair and was able to see and cuddle both my glorious grandsons. We went into lockdown the following week. November, 2020.

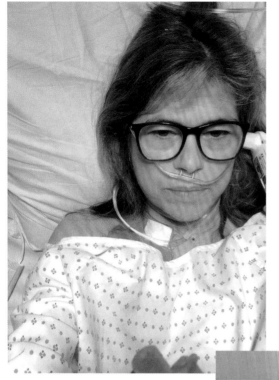

Having just come round from an operation to have my port fitted.

Fully withered, about two months after finishing chemo.

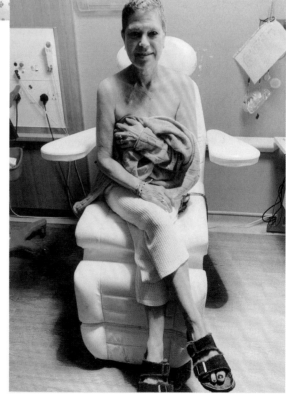

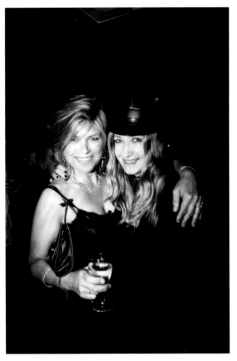

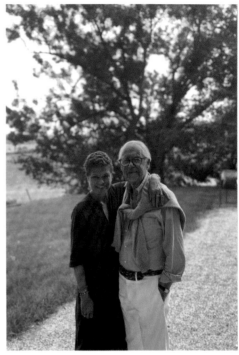

With Anya Hindmarch at a fancy dress party.

Johnnie and me in France, 2022. My Manderley.

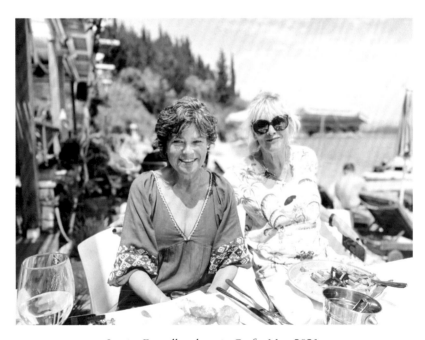

Louise Fennell and me in Corfu. May, 2021.

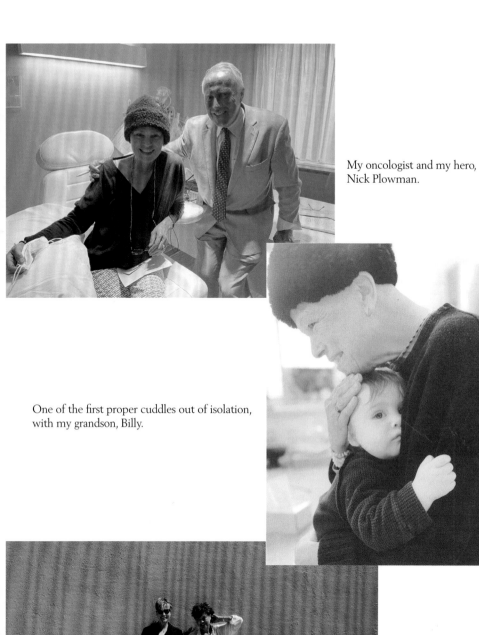

My oncologist and my hero, Nick Plowman.

One of the first proper cuddles out of isolation, with my grandson, Billy.

Sisters – me and Emma. Short hair, don't care.

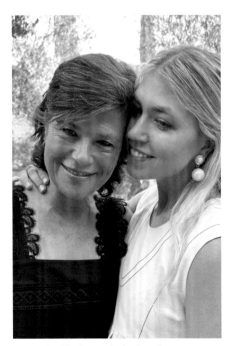

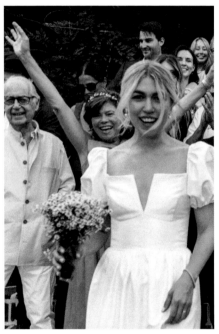

Me and Tills the night before her wedding.

Tilly's wedding to Felix Archer. September, 2022.

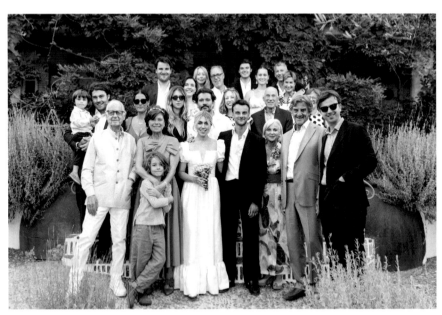

Family affair – the one group wedding photograph we have. Front row: John Standing, me, Huck Thomas, Tilly and Felix, Ruth Archer, Steven Archer, Max Archer. Second row: Archie Standing, Billy, Nisha Grewal, India Standing, Sean Thomas, Aoife O'Donnell, David Warner, Sue Warner. Third row: Josh Archer, Fhionna Redfern, Susie Leon, Alexander Leon, Sam Clempson, Lily Clempson, Graham Clempson and Emma Clempson. The only family member sadly missing was my mum.

the images across a wasteland of deserted London streets.

I text Tilly.

Happy Christmas, darling. Can't wait for our doorstep exchange later.

I know today is going to be a tough one for her. Felix has rightfully gone home to his parents and, although she is in India's bubble, I knew how much Tilly cherishes familiar family traditions, and will be missing them.

Mamma Mia, she texts back. *It's Christmas Day! I've sent you an email. Open it now!!*

I climb back into bed, and switch on my laptop. Open my emails and download a Dropbox video. Press play. Suddenly it is Christmas Day. Tilly has somehow got my family, my friends, my loved-ones all together on a video wishing me a Happy Christmas. They've all dressed up in Abba costumes, accessorised themselves with fairy lights, reindeer antlers; every participating man, woman, child and dog has gone to such an effort. It is totally joyous, and reduces me to floods of tears.

I cry all the time these days. Not out of self-pity. What makes me cry is the kindness that is shown towards me. Cancer not only makes the person going through it appreciate every nuance of life, it also makes the people who love you speak their minds. They put their money where their mouth is. And it's humbling. It may take a village to raise a child, but let me tell you, it takes a gang of past and present friends to instil a future in someone going through the loneliness of having cancer during a pandemic. I watch the video three times on a loop, until I have to take a Nurofen to numb the throbbing, emotional, festive headache I'd given myself.

When Johnnie is awake (and we've watched the video again) we open presents and get dressed. Dressed up. He puts on the new suit he had made a year ago for an important memorial service that was cancelled because of Covid, and I put on the same Lurex trousers I wore to my sixtieth birthday party. 'Go big and stay at home' is my new motto.

We put our patio heater on and spend the morning having individual drive-bys from our three children, sliding presents across the stoop, the weather too cold for us to open them together. Brief encounters.

Hopefully, this apartness will never seem normal. I never want it to. It's alien. Lockdown rules make me think of what it must be like visiting a loved-one in prison. Putting your hand up against a glass barrier, like familiar strangers. Touching but not making contact. We all go through the rituals of love but it's like swimming in treacle. Seeing those you cherish, whilst being unable to physically touch them, is the cruelty of a cock-tease. It's miming to the music with the volume on mute.

Lunch for us on Christmas Day is a Deliveroo pizza. Basic. It arrives two hours late. Johnnie has changed out of his new suit, I've changed back into my pyjamas, and we watch the Queen's speech whilst munching on cold and flaccid Margaritas. It is certainly a different Christmas.

Pathetic, really, how one day in the year can hold such great expectations.

I'm hyper-aware of the potential time bomb of loneliness waiting to explode, faced by all those spending Christmas alone. We've always included waifs and strays in our family celebrations. Christmas Day has only ever been enhanced and improved by the mishmash of people gathered – all ages, from all walks of life – and I can't pretend I don't miss the mayhem.

When it gets dark, Anya and James turn up on our doorstep with delicious home-made plum pudding and brandy butter. Johnnie and I sit on the sofa, just the two of us. Our living room is lit by candles, and we count our blessings.

10

On New Year's Eve I have to go back to hospital for a PET scan, to see how the tumour is reacting to chemo. No great plans for the evening ahead; I know I'll be ready for bed by 8 p.m., having made no resolutions whatsoever, bar staying alive.

Getting dressed in the morning, I put on a sweater I must last have worn at the start of treatment. It is littered with fallen hair; the lone strands clinging like barnacles to the wool. I stare in fascination, before picking them off like scabs. I dream I have hair. I used to have thick, lush, messy hair that I would twizzle up into a clip. Sometimes, instinctively, I go to run my hands through it, but there's nothing there. Apparently, if you lose a limb, you get phantom itching. You still feel a deep connection. I can imagine that. Because at least forty times a day, I reach up towards my scalp, never expecting to touch skin. I am always surprised. It's the convenience of hair I mourn the most, for it goes with everything.

Without it I feel undressed. Unfinished. Invisible. I fanta-sise about standing in the shower and smothering my hair with conditioner, right down to the very ends. Walking about with damp hair turban-wrapped in a thin towel before setting it free and whooshing it dry with my fingers. I can still smell freshly cleaned hair.

And I've become obsessed with eyebrows. My eye-brows. And my eyelashes. They are on the way out. Every member of my family has beautifully defined, thick eye-brows. Even Billy was born with mini McDonald's arches. Archie has thick caterpillars that frame his kind eyes, India's are groomed with that Brooke Shields' insouci-ance, and mine are trained to perfection after years of having them tamed into a perfect arch. Tilly's are the best though. She cut her forehead on a radiator when she was four. I'd gone out to do an early-morning super-market sweep at Sainsbury's and left the children in my bed with Johnnie, watching cartoons. They'd got bored and were mucking about, and Tilly was playing a game with Archie, which entailed her jumping off the bed into his arms. He failed to catch her, as six-year-olds do, and she slammed into the sharp edge of the radiator.

I returned from the shops to find the whole family standing on the pavement. Waiting for me. Ashen. A blood-stained towel was held up against Tilly's eye, and she was cradled in Johnnie's arms.

'Never, ever go to the supermarket in the morning and leave us alone,' he admonished, his panic barely contained. 'Shit happens when you aren't here. Truly.'

I looked under the towel. An open gash. You could see the bone. The doctor didn't stitch it, he glued it, and Tills returned with two little Steri-Strips and a sticker saying, 'I've been brave.' All the ice cream had melted in the boot of my car; cookie dough Häagen-Dazs dripping on to the broccoli and frozen fish fingers I'd bought to have for tea.

Tilly was left with the legacy of a miniature lightning bolt scar cutting through one brow. It's cool. It's like Harry Potter. She wears it with pride.

But I'm personally not quite sure how I'm going to rock the no-brows look. Day by day, they are morphing back into the skimpy, thin, fashionable lines of hair I'd briefly coveted in the seventies. Plucked within an inch of their lives; a mean brow that was all the rage back then. And my lashes have become very sparse. They are like a newborn's. Like a baby's, fresh out of the womb.

The PET scan necessitates being injected with some radioactive liquid and having my glucose levels tested an hour before going into the tunnel.

'How are you feeling?' my oncologist asked last week.

'Okay,' I replied. 'I feel okay. I mean, I accept, I do feel totally wiped out and fragile, but I'm guessing that's to be expected. I feel like I've been forced to accept this time bomb within me. It's blasting off and everything is imploding. It's not an option any more. It's happening.' I get it. Sadly.

'I'm afraid I rate facts more than feelings,' he said

apologetically. 'I like looking at reality. Results. Data. Not really impressed by the rest.'

This is exactly why I like him so much. He has one mission, and one mission only: to get me out of this mess. Sympathy ain't going to work. But hopefully medicine is.

This is my second PET scan. I know from experience the patient is always asked if they suffer from claustrophobia. Luckily, I don't. In fact, I find this test quite relaxing. I imagine I'm in a spaceship, because unlike other machine-led tests, it's conducted in silence. I lie poker straight, a plastic support under my knees, my body wrapped in a blanket, and internally I sing Bowie's 'Space Oddity' to myself.

> Far above the world
> Planet Earth is blue
> And there's nothing I can do.

The lyrics resonate. There is a feeling of acceptance when you're given a cancer diagnosis. There is nothing you can do, bar deal with it. You can't roll the dice hoping for a different outcome. It's there. It's got you. You can't cheat. You can't put it on the back burner, or hope it will just go away. It's got into your DNA, and like a creepy space invader it's set up lodgings. The only way out is to put your trust in science. To do as you are told. The world seems a very different place when you arrive at this conclusion. Indeed, planet Earth is blue. Choices removed, decisions made, predestined timetables drawn up. It makes you both supremely selfish and at the same time totally compliant. Like a child having to fit in with its parents' schedule.

I find the selfishness manifests itself in what little control I have left over my life. I do as I like. Sleep when I feel like it, eat what I want, get emotional when I can't stop myself. I exist within my own parameters and follow my own body clock. I'm raw. I'm not dissimilar to my ten-month-old grandson, Billy, who hasn't yet learnt the art of fitting into the conventions that society demands of him. We're both at the wanton, virgin, exploratory stage of discovery. He's busy figuring out how to crawl, how to open shut cupboards, and seeing if he likes the taste of courgettes over carrots. He is often indifferent to any routine. He finds joy in every dawn, regardless of the broken sleep he's inflicted on his poor parents.

Whilst he's learning how to live his new life, I'm learning how to adapt my new life to the old life I once had. Both of us are wearing our emotions on our sleeves and both of us are hard-wired to rage against imagined injustices. He throws himself on to the floor when prevented from getting hold of the television controls. I lean up against a wall and hit it when I find myself too weak to walk as far, or as fast, as I'd planned. We are both railing and wailing. I just happen to do most of mine silently. I embarrass myself.

For the first time in my adult life, all major decisions have been made for me. I'm a baby, back to having a set routine.

Morning pill-taking. Then my stats. Blood pressure, temperature, pulse, oxygen levels.

Eat breakfast. 'Good girl, you've got a clean plate.' This makes Johnnie happy.

Drink. Drink. Drink. Water. Water. Water. Hydrate.

Bath time. Check that the water isn't too hot, because chemo skin is sensitive. Dry properly in all the cracks, because, like little Billy, you can get chafed patches easily.

Get dressed. Put on an ugly vest, to keep warm.

All this activity is a bit exhausting, so I lie down for an hour and reboot my energy. Only, unlike Billy, I don't fight a mid-morning nap.

I mooch about, playing with my toys. Fisher-Price replaced by iPhone, laptop, *The Times* newspaper and Radio 4.

I hydrate. Again.

A slow walk around the block. A very slow walk. Mask on, gloves on, hat on, scarf, coat. I need a mother to layer me up against the cold and insist that I wear my thermals.

Lunch. I don't really want to eat lunch. Not hungry.

'You must eat, darling,' says Johnnie gently. 'Have a bit more.'

Compliance. But nothing tastes good with metal mouth. It's like eating after a root canal treatment. My tongue is numb and there is a pervading film of stannic-like yuckiness that rules supreme over any other flavour. Nothing I try succeeds in overriding it. I have to accept that I am going to spoon spinach and water-cress soup down my throat as though I'm swallowing unpleasant-tasting medicine. India makes me a fresh delivery twice a week. Neon green. She adds the spinach at the last minute so it keeps its colour.

Johnnie is extremely attentive towards me; we've temporarily reversed roles. As the much younger wife, I've always assumed the role of caretaker in the past. It was easy. Because I was hardly ever ill.

Now he's filling hot-water bottles, making me cups of tea, going out to buy the newspapers, endlessly unloading the dishwasher, emptying the rubbish, rubbing my feet, making my bed comfy. Sweetly doing jigsaws he has no interest in doing. Watching TV programmes he doesn't really want to watch, to keep me company. Offering to cook me dinner. I can't accept too many of Johnnie's culinary attempts, as they all revolve around eggs. Omelettes, scrambled, fried, boiled. On rotation. But it's the thought that counts. And normally I love eggs. Just not every day.

It's a wildly sweeping statement, but in my experience, I've discovered most actors are totally ill-equipped to deal with real life. I think it's probably one of the main reasons they become actors in the first place. They exist in a sort of arrested state of development and are child-like in their stubborn reluctance to engage with the normal, everyday hiccups of house maintenance. Parking permits, form-filling, booking travel tickets, changing light bulbs that are high up in the ceiling, turning a router on and off to reboot the internet. Mending or fixing almost anything, in fact.

They've never experienced the daily grind of a regular

nine to five job. No actor in the world is fortunate enough to be gainfully employed for forty-nine weeks of the year, not even if they are starring in a soap opera or are a world-famous film star. The majority jog along, do a job, get paid and then enjoy a break whilst endlessly bugging their agents for another job. On set, on location, or in the theatre, they have dressers to dress them. Make-up artists to transform them into different characters. Drivers to drive them. Assistants to bring them cups of coffee and lunch. Their life is organised by other people. Nannied. They are taken care of in order to be free to act.

I remember Johnnie once shouting at me when we had a massive leak gushing through the ceiling and I was instructing him to turn the water off at the mains, 'Darling, you married an actor, not a plumber. What on earth makes you think I would know where the mains are?'

They are, however, brilliant at many other things: playing imaginative games with children, reading bedside stories with lots of different voices, having an infectiously laissez-faire attitude towards authority, and ensuring that life in their presence is never, not even for a split second, dull or boring.

When actors are between jobs they like to say they are 'resting'. Never unemployed. Resting. It may financially be a hand-to-mouth existence at times, true feast or famine, but I've never known anything else. Or loved a lifestyle more. Dramatic at times, sometimes scary. But I wouldn't swap the delirious joy of never knowing what possible fortunes are waiting around the corner for a measured existence. It keeps me on my toes, and life can never be accused of being mundane.

But are actors in general – or Johnnie in particular – equipped with the tools of a full-time carer and house husband? Not so much.

But he is trying extremely hard, and I love him dearly for it.

I miss my mum terribly. She lives at least an hour away and no longer drives, which means she can't even come and stand on my doorstep. I don't know how she's coping with me being ill and her living alone. It haunts me that I can't see her.

Once, a friend kindly drove her up to London and I opened the kitchen window wide so the room was Siberian cold. We sat twenty feet apart from each other, eating a bowl of soup, mutually way too nervous to get any closer. Each too scared we might infect the other. Cold comforts. I can't imagine how hard this must be for her. She took three photographs of me, from a distance, like a souvenir.

I talk to my sister in New York relentlessly on Face-Time. She props up the phone in her kitchen and we just chew the fat aimlessly whilst both doing nothing. We agree we are both desperate housewives, up to very little, living countries apart, separated by a lockdown pandemic. But the normality of talking to her grounds me. I need her. I need our shared history. I need our shorthand; I crave the normality of our history. I need to know the minutiae of her day-to-day existence. I just ache to be in the same room as her, and this is as good as it's going to get right now.

She's very good at going with my flow. Picking up my rhythms. She doesn't tell me how I ought to be feeling. She knows me too well – and anyway, I'm six years older than she, so she wouldn't dare tell me what to do, even now. I've been the trailblazer all our lives; the rule-breaker, the naughty one, the defiant one, the risk-taker. And cancer hasn't changed my attitude. Not one jot. Emma accepts me, and I adore her for that. She bombards me with weekly FedEx-ed care packages. They arrive on my doorstep like love letters. Full of warm hats, chewing gum to combat my dry mouth, perhaps a new pair of pyjamas, a trashy book, a kaftan she found and knows I'd like to wear on future summer holidays spent together. Rewards for the fact I'm halfway towards a return to normality. A sisterly star chart.

She doesn't demand I live up to any expectations. I sometimes find that friends want to infuse someone they care about with exhausting optimism. They are probably at a loss for what to say. And they want me to feel better. So they park their fears – too close to home, perhaps? – and put all their money on well-intentioned platitudes.

'You've got this,' they say with absolute certainty. 'If anyone can cope with this, it's you. Cancer picked the wrong person to fuck with. You *are* going to come through this. I have no doubt in my mind whatsoever. You will sail through this and come out the other side.

My friend had the identical same cancer as you, and that was twenty-five years ago. You've got this. Trust me.'

Fighting words like that panic me. No lie. They fill me with fear. Because they leave no room for a margin of medical error. I'm a born people pleaser. I never want to let people down. I don't like to appear vulnerable, or to ask for help. Sometimes their words play back to me on repeat, just before I go to sleep at night. A nasty, incessant niggle. A gremlin of doubt that plagues me.

Because what if I don't have this? What if I'm too broken to mend in the way everyone wants me to mend? What if I don't snap back to being optimistic and carefree? What if I find darkness where before I only saw light? What if this treatment throws me an unexpected curve ball and doesn't comply with the timelines? It can, might and could well happen. What if I'm too fatigued to go back to work full-time?

What if? What if? What if?

What if I fail?

What if I don't make it?

What if I die and disappoint you?

I don't ever want to let everyone down.

I shut my mind down at this point. Gag it. I will myself to take a leaf out of my oncologist's book and rate facts above feelings.

The scan results have come back and he is 'pleased' with them. Everything is 'progressing nicely'.

I must continue to look forward and remember that tomorrow is another day.

11

Every day I must adjust to a new exterior. A new body. I've completely lost my bottom. Gone. It used to be quite perky for my age. Now it's had the stuffing sucked out of it, a combination of uncontrolled weight loss and a lack of exercise. I used to look at middle-aged women wearing trousers that fitted around their waist but had too much fabric dangling around their arse and be grateful that mine still clung to my buttocks. Those halcyon days are over. My cushion has gone. Flat butt. All this body morphing is nothing short of weird. No part of my body remains familiar territory. I can (and do) try to maintain a semblance of normality by putting on make-up, but I feel like an actor playing a part.

I mention this to my therapist. I've never seen a therapist before. The hospital gives me the option to have a session of reflexology or an hour with their therapist to while away the time during chemo. To help with the avalanche of feelings and emotions. I normally opt for reflexology because my feet are permanently painful, and I consider myself fine. Coping. But today the reflexologist can't see me, so I decide to go for the therapy on offer. Out of curiosity more than any need. She's called Susie and she's nervous. Or maybe I make her nervous. She scurries in and presses herself against the wall opposite my bed.

'Is this a good time?' she asks.

'Sure,' I reply, snapping my laptop closed. I am three seasons into watching *How to Get Away with Murder* and am totally hooked. This is not a good time.

Susie cocks her head to one side, which makes her mask and visor go comically askew. I note that she has a white streak of hair either side of her ears, not unlike a racoon, and is wearing Crocs with blue socks. This is the problem with being a writer. You notice things too much and have an innate desire to ask questions.

'How are you coping?' she enquires.

'Okay, I think,' I say. 'Good. I mean I seem to be handling the chemo. I haven't been sick, or anything like that, so far. And I'm so bloody grateful I haven't had to deal with that.'

'Grateful,' says Susie. 'Interesting.'

My choice of adjective hangs in the air between us like an insult.

'Well, yes,' I reply. 'I hate feeling sick more than anything else in the world. So I am grateful.'

'Really?'

I'm no good at this. I don't do literal speak, and I realise that Susie is pecking. She's pecking over every word I utter like a hen looking for corn kernels on a barren patch of grass. I like bold words. Why use 'dislike' when one could use 'hate', 'pleased' when 'bloody grateful' is more effective? I get both bold and bored. And feisty.

'I find I care more about how my treatment affects the other people in my life, rather than how it affects me,' I say, throwing out a mini hand grenade of self-awareness for Susie to work with.

'Ah. Very interesting,' she says. 'Do you find that applies to other aspects of your life as well?'

'No.'

This conversation is going absolutely nowhere, and I really want to get back to watching Viola Davis on Netflix. So, in order to speed things up, I start asking Susie questions. It's so much easier. And anyway, it's what I used to do in my previous life as a journalist.

'How long have you worked in the hospital?' I ask, manoeuvring my bed into an upright position. 'Did you always want to be a therapist dealing with cancer patients?'

And she's off and running. Her mother had breast cancer and Susie decided it would be lovely to give something back, so she started working in a hospice dealing with end-of-life patients. After three years, she found she was becoming emotionally drained, so she switched from palliative care to talking to those undergoing treatment for cancer. And she was going to the Maldives for Christmas. Looking forward to it.

I could start a discussion about how I think it's morally wrong to travel during a pandemic, but I don't. I can't be bothered. Instead, I tell her how wonderful snorkelling is in the sea there. And how, when I went, I fed stingrays. Who make a strange snorting sound when they ground themselves on the beach.

'If you have any concerns before our next session, you can always email me. You know that, don't you?' says Susie sweetly, gathering up her notes.

'I do,' I reply. 'I will. I hope you have a lovely holiday.'

I can see I'm a lousy contender for therapy, although I totally appreciate how it can be a lifeline for some. I've never been good at self-examination, or interested in searching through the detritus stored in the attic of my past. Perhaps having a truly happy childhood offers some sort of protection against self-doubt. Or maybe it's just that I lack the concentration required to search for the answers to questions I've never taken the time to ask.

During my first encounter with Susie, she asks if I think I might be suffering from post-traumatic stress disorder: seeing as how I went from seeing a specialist to being diagnosed with cancer in under eight hours.

I think about it for a few moments and briefly entertain the fact that she might be on to something. And then I dismiss it.

'But if I was, surely that would indicate I'm in denial?' I ask. 'And I'm not. I know I've got cancer. I accept that.

And I realise I must have treatment. And I'm just glad I got diagnosed so quickly and didn't have to wait for weeks to find out what was wrong with me.'

Deep, deep down I knew something wasn't right. And I beat myself up over that. Like coming to the end of a love affair, it's so tempting to ignore the warning signs and to postpone the descent of the final curtain. To disregard the niggly little intrusions, rather than examining them collectively and raising the red flag of concern. For me, the straw that broke my personal camel's back was being too breathless to pick Billy up.

Why was I so oblivious? Why did I disregard the signs? What does it matter? Who knows? Who cares? I can't trawl backwards through time and rewrite history. What's the point in discussing PTSD? It doesn't change my outcome.

The only way out of cancer is to move forwards. And I want out.

I also now want out of hospital in the fastest possible time. The dreaded second strain of Covid has struck and it's not a wave, it's a tsunami. We're back in full lockdown.

When I went to the hospital to have my bloods taken two days ago, before having my third round of chemo today, everything had changed. For the first time I no longer felt safe.

On the ground floor of the hospital, there was a lot of action. Everyone was scurrying about in full PPE, as opposed to just masks and gloves, and the safety precautions for patients had tightened.

'You are going to a different floor for your bloods today,' I was informed when I checked in. 'Not oncology. Your nurse will meet you at the lift.'

And Lena did meet me. Double masked, visored up, aproned and gloved, opening the swing doors with her elbow. No hands.

'It's bad,' she said as she tightened the rubber tourniquet around my upper arm, and seamlessly started to draw phial after phial of blood into mini glass bottles.

'We've been told with this new strain that we should avoid talking to patients, even if we are both wearing masks. Unless we are six feet away. Particles can get through masks made damp through talking. Obviously, there are certain times we must,' she said, shrugging and pulling out the long stick used to swab my throat for Covid.

I held my breath as much as I could with my mouth wide open. Lena stepped quickly away from me.

'It really scares me,' I said. 'How often do all of you get tested?'

'Twice a week,' she replied. 'And obviously, if anyone tests positive, we have to stay home and isolate. But don't you worry, all the Covid patients are up on a separate floor. They're not on the chemo ward.'

But I do worry. Selfishly, I do. I can't help it. I'm simply terrified of catching Covid in hospital. I imagine I can control my home environment, for I barely leave my house, except to take exercise. I let fresh air in every day and insist all deliveries are left on the doorstep. I wear rubber gloves to unpack them. I am careful.

When Johnnie and I go out for a walk, we act like Russian spies. We walk at a fair pace, my eyes darting from side to side, observing who is coming towards us. If they are unmasked, we both cross the street. If someone seems to be following too closely, I walk faster in order to distance myself. I take no risks. Because chemo annihilates the immune system, I am – not unsurprisingly – paranoid about germs.

Throughout my diagnosis, tests, biopsies, scans and first two sessions of chemo I was lucky. Covid cases in this country were relatively stable. Hospitals were coping. Now they've gone into free fall. The country is bracing itself for the onslaught.

I vow that however crap I feel, this time I'm going to go home the second the Red Devil infusion is in me. So, I've brought my own pillow to the hospital. And I've repacked my chemo bag with antiseptic wipes, my hand sanitiser, masks and gloves.

Today I lie fully dressed on the bed, with my own blanket from home covering me. I wipe down the side of the table and the buzzer. When the nurse sets up the infusion stand, I ask what I should do if I need to pee whilst attached to it. I don't want to call for help. I want to minimise any contact.

'You just disconnect the green plug at the back,' she says, showing me. 'Do your thing, and then replug yourself in when you're done.'

I lie very still and watch the various bags slowly emptying their contents into my line. I need to pee. I unplug.

I am the most uncoordinated member of my family. I can't dance. Well, obviously I can, but I dance to the beat of a very different drum. A drum that isn't actually the one being played. In my mind, I'm a wicked combination of Michael Jackson and Madonna, whereas in reality I'm like the rogue drunk uncle at a family wedding out to impress. The one everyone tries to distance themselves from as he enthusiastically takes to the floor. My family tease me about it. Because I have no rhythm. None. I admit it. Reluctantly. Things improve slightly after I've downed a couple of vodka shots, but barely. I just get bolder and become impervious to my own lack of talent. I often do a solo turn. Needs must.

But my infusion stand turns out to be my perfect dance partner. Who knew? Silent, steady and extremely compliant. Unjudgemental. I disconnect my stand from the wall and grab it by its skinny little stick waist. I glide across the floor, deftly spinning it to untangle the snaking tubes in order to avoid air bubbles and kinks. I waltz into the bathroom like a gazelle and position my stand next to me as I lower myself on to the loo, keeping one hand firmly on my now stationary dance partner. Up I get, and we're off again.

Dancing with the Red Devil. Smooth moves. *Cha-cha-cha!*

I do one final twirl, before reconnecting my partner to the wall, and flop back on to the bed.

My body may be changing beyond all recognition but there is hope on the horizon. Two days after completing round three, and still high on steroids, I go off to Wimpole Street to finally collect my wig. Because it's bespoke, and not something flammable I've ordered online from Amazon, it has to be fitted and adjusted in situ. Tweaked. This is a medical wig facility that caters only for patients who have lost their hair through illness, so is allowed to continue operating during lockdown restrictions.

Temperature taken, full PPE worn, and a clear Covid test before admission.

I wind my way down a narrow staircase and wait in a basement room kitted out like a private room at a hairdresser's. I sit alone in front of the mirror and look at myself. I'm wearing a bright pink knitted beanie and have put make-up on.

I wear a beanie 24/7, including when I'm in bed. I Skype my six-year-old, highly observant grandson most mornings. Never once has Huck noticed or questioned why I'm wearing a hat in bed, nor has he queried where my hair has gone. India and I keep bracing ourselves for the question, but it never comes. We are exceptionally close, Hucky and I, and when we used to snuggle in bed at night with our heads close together, reading stories, our hair colour and texture were interchangeable. People often used to say he'd inherited my hair. Since I got ill, he's inexplicably refused to cut his, despite his mother's best efforts. He's grown a thick mane, just as I've lost mine. A mini Hugh Grant bouffant of lushness and wanton messiness. He now has to grab a big handful and push it out of his eyes whenever he talks to me. His hair both transfixes and obsesses me. The irony is not lost on me – it's as though my loss has become his gain, and taken up temporary residence on his head. My little hirsute doppelgänger.

'Hello, my darling,' says Jackie, my wig-maker, bursting into the room with what looks like a flat, Disney princess sea of hair balanced on one fist.

I look at this three-foot-long freedom pass she's holding out before me. It's not what I'm expecting. It's sort of terrifying.

'I think the colour is a bit brassy compared to the samples you sent me of your own hair, don't you?' she asks. 'I'm going to pop next door and quickly apply a toner. I'll bring the radio in so you can listen to it while you're waiting. Then we can try the wig on, adjust the tension if I need to, and you'll be ready for your hairdresser to cut it.'

Clive. Clive, my saviour, has arrived, also kitted out in PPE, to cut and style my sheitel. I had momentarily forgotten I was having it cut. If anyone can kill the fisted Disney princess, it's Clive. I trust him implicitly to recreate my own personality.

Jackie returns with my slightly damp, toned-down hair on one hand. It reminds me of a ventriloquist's dummy, only I'm the bald (as opposed to fat) controller. Once it's on my head, I'm going to bring it to life.

On it goes. Jackie and Clive both stare at it.

'Her hairline is slightly further back,' instructs Clive who has been looking at me in the mirror for over thirty years.

Jackie makes a minute tug.

'That's it.'

'Does it feel secure?' asks Jackie, grabbing the hidden band of elastic beneath my neck. 'Or is that better?'

'Um, maybe that's better,' I reply.

'I'll be right back,' says Jackie, carefully removing my locks. 'Quick adjustment.'

Clive and I stare at my bald head.

'How long did my cut last?' he asks.

'Two days,' I reply sadly. 'And then my parting widened and I got tufts. I looked like a cancer victim with a comb-over. I got them to shave it at the hospital.'

'Well, I can tell you now,' says Clive, 'I've dealt with lots of clients who have lost their hair through chemo. But I've never encountered anyone whose hair came out as fiercely as yours. I didn't want to say anything at the time, but it was like cutting quicksand.'

My eyes prick with tears as I remember that night. 'Do you think you will be able to do something with the wig?'

'Your wig is fab-u-lous,' he replies. 'Trust me. By the

time I've finished with you, you won't know the difference.'

Once it's back in situ, he starts spritzing it down, just like old times. He cuts, he flicks, he sections it off.

Snip, snip, snip.

The floor becomes littered with discarded hair. I relax and just let him get on with it.

'I'm going to leave the fringe a bit longer, so it hides your eyebrows.'

'Whatever you think,' I reply.

He stands back to admire his work before plugging in his hairdryer.

Ten minutes later, I'm looking at myself in the mirror. My real self. My internal playlist jump-starts: Michael Jackson.

If you wanna make the world a better place
Take a look at yourself and then make a change.

I need to accept myself. The new me. I need to change.

Goodbye, pity party. I now have hair. Have hair, don't care. I stuff my beanie into my handbag, thank Clive and Jackie, and leave the building with a swish in my step. My hair flutters in the wind.

Postscript: I wear the wig exactly twice. It requires a lot of fiddly fixing. It is a high-maintenance mop. It needs tape. A tightened band around my scalp to make it stable. It's a faff. It's surprisingly heavy. And despite the fact it has been meticulously dyed to supposedly match my own hair colour, it doesn't. It's dark. It's lifeless. An imposter. Vaguely like my own hair. But not. Like a dark, coiffed wig in fact.

Three days after leaving with a swish in my step and hair fluttering in the wind, I decide I hate it.

Four days later, a friend of mine from America sends me a present. Soft thermals, some CBD gummies, some plastic trucks to give to Billy, and what looks like a merkin in a gauze bag. I open it gingerly, not quite knowing what to expect. It is a wig. *Something to give you a laugh*, Rita has written on the note. *You can play around with it.*

It is a slip-on. Short. Blond. Light as a feather. I try it. For a laugh. I wear it in the same way I'd wear a hat. I plonk it on with zero aplomb. And zero expectations. It is love at first sight. It makes me look completely different, as opposed to an inferior, look-alike version of myself. I subsequently google the brand and find they come from a website called www.simplywigs.co.uk and are available in England. I shop the Raquel Welch collection. Auburn, dark. Short, shorter.

I put a post on Instagram saying if anyone has lost their hair through chemo or alopecia and wants a 'barely worn wig' made from human hair, I will happily donate mine. First come, first served.

A lovely woman who is terminally ill with cancer and receiving palliative care replies, saying she hates being bald, has long ago lost all confidence, and her greatest wish is to die in a wig.

Her partner emails me not long after I've sent it. He says she wore my wig to the bitter end.

Paying it forward.

Like a scene from a Victorian novel, I made my father a promise on his deathbed. I really did. I promised that I would always take care of my mother, and now I've broken that promise. For six years I've honoured his dying wishes, and now I physically can't. I haven't even laid eyes on her for seven long weeks. I last saw her at the beginning of December, when she drove all the way up from Windlesham to stand on my doorstep in the freezing cold for ten minutes. The distance between us is both unnatural and acute. I find it unbearable. Sadness runs through my body like letters in a stick of Brighton rock.

When I was little, my mother always made my birthday cakes. Back in the good old days when children's parties were all about paper hats and eating eggy sandwiches, cocktail sausages, and lurid orange jelly set in individual flower-shaped moulds. Cake was always the celebratory climax, gobbled up before climbing down from the table and running off to play Musical Chairs and Pass the Parcel.

I can remember all my cakes with the utmost clarity. A train one year. A clock, with a little mouse running up it. A farm, studded with a fence made of Cadbury's chocolate fingers, and my lead pigs and cows pushed down into the green-grass icing. Every creation festooned with Smarties, their colour slightly bleeding out at the edges. The ceremonial lighting of the candles, the singing of

'Happy Birthday'. I remember it all. My mother holding my long hair back from my face as I blew, my chubby cheeks inflated with pleasure. And then the wish. I always made the same wish. Always. Back in those glorious, innocent days – the time before I really understood the concept of mortality. I made the same wish every year. I wished my parents would live forever.

My mother has managed to fulfil my childhood yearning, for sixty-one years. Unlike me, she has kept her promise. A widow after fifty-nine years of marriage; she is now isolated. Not only through her ongoing grief, but also through lockdown. The double whammy. Her days are no longer punctuated by visits from friends and family. Hers are lonely, long days, uninterrupted by sharing a life with my dad. Emma and I have tried our best to fill the chasm he left behind. But in truth we only partially succeed – in the way an incurable leak can only be temporarily stemmed. According to the dictionary, loneliness is an emotional response to perceived isolation. Except this nationwide isolation isn't perceived. It's real.

She's my mother and yet she can't care for me. That destroys both of us. I am never too old for my mother's reassuring touch. She belongs to a generation that is instinctively predisposed to fear, mistrust and question medicine and the miracles of science. I understand. I think children brought up during the war had low expectations of cures and medical interventions.

Cancer was whisperingly referred to as 'the C word' and spoken as an expletive, a stain on one's character. It was secretive; almost shameful. Both my mother's parents died ridiculously young by today's standards, yet their exact cause of death is hazy. Fuzzy. Their medical treatment, as remembered by my mother, was 'terrifying'. And back in the fifties, I'm sure she was right.

I think back to how basic our childhood medicine cabinet was, and what my sister and I were given when we were ill. Milk of Magnesia for upset tummies, the blue glass bottle of thick, chalky liquid we had to choke down, and which inexplicably always left a tiny line of white residue on our lips. Vick's Vapour Rub for bad chests, the greasiness and smell of camphor sticking to our flannel nighties. Weird, squiggly brown granules in a sachet that tasted of dehydrated chocolate, for constipation; and dissolvable, bitter aspirin, for fevers. I remember my mother warming up olive oil (in those days bought at the chemist's) whenever we had an earache, and soaking a piece of cotton wool in it before placing it, soothingly, in the affected ear. It provided warmth, comfort and temporary relief. Iglodine ointment for bloodied knees. It stung, and we had to wait for it to dry before our wound was covered with fabric Elastoplast.

Most fondly, I remember Haliborange tablets. Tiny pills that were sour, but in a good way. Emma and I loved them and would frequently self-medicate. They were a one-a-day vitamin for children, given throughout winter, to stave off colds. But to us, they were like crack. As addictive as our once-a-day treat from the sweetie jar after lunch. The acidity made your tongue rough, like a cat's lick, and when unsupervised we would binge on them. Sucking off the outer coating then crunching them up.

Being poorly when I was little was a big, bedridden event. Everyday routine was put on hold. Pillows plumped, hot-water bottles filled, trays of food delivered. Mummy was an amazing nurse. She would place cold, wet, wrung-out facecloths on our foreheads, read to us, play board games if we felt well enough, and bring up plates of tempting food. Scrambled eggs with buttery toast and a dollop of tomato ketchup; a little bunch of grapes and a Petit Suisse with a sprinkling of sugar. Ribena and digestive biscuits for tea. If we felt any better after a midday nap, we were allowed to snuggle up in slippers and a dressing gown and see *Watch with Mother*: Bill and Ben, Andy Pandy or the Woodentops were our favourites. Daddy would pop in throughout the day, if he was at home working, and lie on my bed for a few minutes and stroke my arm and make up stories. If I was properly ill and feverish, Mummy would sleep with me.

I loved all that.

What, perversely, I love about having cancer during lockdown is the way it's made me rediscover time. Now I actually enjoy the yawning expanse of hours stretching ahead of me. After forty years of adhering to a fairly rigid, structured life determined by routine, deadlines and schedules, I really like the experience of going into meandering free fall. Cancer has pushed me off the treadmill. And I'm grateful for that in a way I never anticipated.

In my old life I was always in a mad rush to reach my destination. It was like travelling on a high-speed train. Hurry, hurry, hurry. When trains go fast, and you look out of the window, you see flashing tableaux of life. They whizz past like snapshots from television programmes on fast forward. Glimpses. Fragments. Another platform. Another station. A field. An industrial estate. A back garden. A tunnel. A town. Catch it if you can.

My life was like that. Don't get me wrong; I loved it. But I now realise I allowed it to go by so fast. Way too fast. I seldom stopped to reflect; too busy craning my neck to catch sight of the next vista opening up before me.

Now I've been forced to get on the slow train. I'm no longer worrying about arriving on time at my destination. Miraculously, I'm enjoying the journey itself. It's a revelation. For the first time in a long while, it's as if I'm looking out of the window at the laundry hanging on the line, the little allotments, the cluster of lambs, the wind-torn village bunting left flapping on a post. I'm not functioning on fast forward any more. I'm now watching the programme of my life unfold in real time. And I sort of want to invest in a return ticket. I'm getting used to the pace.

I've become surprisingly used to living in slow motion. I remember, as a child, how time used to stand still at the start of the summer holidays. They would stretch and yawn before me, merging into one blurry haze of carefree abandon.

I feel like that again. Untethered. It's sort of fabulous.

*

Summer holidays offered very little agenda for us as kids. Because both my parents were in the film industry, we didn't really adhere to the standard middle-class conventions of pre-planned summer holidays. If my father was making a film abroad, Emma and I always went with him, often for extended periods of time. Both my parents believed that staying together as a family was paramount. We went to a local school, or when that wasn't practical, we were tutored.

I was just five when I was enrolled in a new school in America. It was 1965, and my father was directing a Hollywood film for Columbia Pictures called *King Rat*. My mother was pregnant with my sister and suffering horrendously from prolonged morning sickness. She later told me she was prescribed pills by her American obstetrician that, fortuitously, she threw away. It was a good call. They turned out to be Thalidomide.

We lived in a rented, modern, Jetsons-style bungalow high up in the hills of Laurel Canyon. Back in the sixties the air really was perfumed by orange blossom. The view from our hilltop at night was picture-perfect, undimmed by the insidious smog that now, sadly, smothers the city below. It was like fairyland; shimmering and blurring beneath the huge night sky. We had a curvy pool that lit up, and I could see its alluring fluorescent glow through my bedroom curtains at night. Three blow-up, oversized swans floated on the surface (decades before Taylor Swift Instagrammed herself having summer fun on a giant inflatable), and I remember I used to check religiously that they were still there in the morning when I awoke. I was obsessed by those swans.

I was taught to swim properly, by an instructor. Not namby-pamby breast strokes, but a strong crawl. And the art of doing a little jump before diving. My mother would wind my long hair into a topknot and wrestle it into a rubber swimming cap festooned with multicoloured rubber flowers. I had a pink bikini bottom that was frilled at the back, and I would be greased up with Coppertone sun lotion every morning before being set free to swim. I spent hours and hours swimming. My mother shielded herself on a sunlounger beside the pool, always holding a tissue or a towel up to her mouth in an attempt (I now realise) to avoid getting that weird brown 'mask of pregnancy' that the sun can activate. I went nut brown and freckled that summer; diving in and out of the pool like a yo-yo. Driving my mother insane with my endless pleas – 'Watch, Mummy, watch. Watch this one!' – before eventually being cajoled out of my mermaid existence. Skin wrinkled and dehydrated by the chlorine, my hair damp and sticking to my scalp when released from the vice-like pressure of my swimming cap.

I adored everything America had to offer. I think, on reflection, this was the turning point for my parents' fortunes; although I was very young and oblivious to their newfound wealth. This film was my dad's big Hollywood break, and whilst he was off filming on a vast set built on a desert wasteland, my mum and I were off having fun in sunny California. We'd visit the set often. I'd always been taken on to sets and locations, ever since I was a toddler, so I knew the drill. The minute the first assistant shouted, 'All quiet, cameras rolling,' followed by my dad saying, 'And action,' I had to stand stock-still, hardly breathing, remaining totally silent, until he said, 'Cut!' I don't know why he always said 'and action', not just 'action', but that has always stayed with me. His total concentration, absorbed in the scene he was directing. Focusing on the actors.

He used to give me little cameos in his films. A good luck mascot. Not in *King Rat*, as it was an all-male cast, but I remember the first time he did. I was two years old, and he was filming one of the penultimate scenes in his directorial debut, *Whistle Down the Wind*. I had on a Paddington Bear blue duffle coat, and my fat little legs were stuffed into a pair of tiny wellington boots. It was the scene where Alan Bates is led out of the barn and arrested by the police, and all the village children have lined up in protest as they (wrongly) assume his character to be Jesus Christ, whereas in reality he was a murderer. It's an incredibly moving scene. And it was a complicated one to shoot, as it involved a long, panning shot lasting about ninety seconds, taking in every child's face. I was at the end of the line, holding hands with an older girl.

'And action,' said Daddy.

The camera rolled and duly moved slowly from the barn, scanning every face, until it stopped at me.

'Hello, Daddy,' I belted out as he passed me on the cherry-picker crane. 'Whatcha doing up there?'

Scene aborted. Followed by a rather terse, 'Cut!'

In America, on afternoons when we weren't visiting the set, my mother would take me to Will Wright's Ice Cream Parlor, on the corner of Beverly Drive and Charleville Boulevard, after school. We'd drive down Laurel Canyon in an open-top car, the radio blasting out 'Baby Love' by the Supremes.

I remember standing inside the cool, air-conditioned, pink and white palace of icy delights and staring up at the billboard-sized menu. My mum would read it out to me.

'Now, do you want peach parfait, mint chocolate chip, raspberry ripple, rocky road or peppermint twist?' she'd ask.

'Vanilla,' I'd reply. Always vanilla. Safe vanilla.

And back we'd climb into the car, leatherette seats boiled by the relentless sun. The backs of my bare legs sticking to the upholstery like glue, the melting ice cream dripping on to my thighs.

Every weekday, I'd put on my uniform, grab my tin lunch box and be taken down the hill to wait for the yellow school bus that would deliver me to Berkeley School. I don't remember being remotely daunted by this huge step away from the comforts of home. I think perhaps my confidence came from being an only child for a large chunk of my childhood. So much of my time was spent playing alone, coupled with the fact I was a naturally gregarious little girl, so I think I probably just loved being part of a gang. A new gang.

Don't forget, I also belonged to the generation whose parents relied on *Dr Spock's Baby and Child Care* as a manual to guide them through the maze of child-rearing. A revered American paediatrician, Dr Spock had his feet placed firmly on the ground. 'To parent' was not considered a verb, back in the day, and 'parenting' was yet to be declared an art. It was a simpler journey; less fraught with self-doubt and complications. One got pregnant, gave birth and became a parent. In the sixties children were both seen and heard, but parents weren't yet held hostage to the capricious whims of their off-spring. Children fitted in with their parents' lives, as opposed to parents kowtowing to their children's needs. Goals consisted of successful weaning; early potty train-ing to end the tyranny of terrycloth nappies soaking in buckets of Napisan; forced afternoon naps for us kids, taken until it was time to start primary school; eating everything on our plate if we wanted pudding (because of the starving and less fortunate); and an insistence on good manners.

I liked my new school. The only day I didn't like it was the day I wet myself whilst in assembly. We were all sitting cross-legged on the shiny wooden floor, with our teachers standing in front of us. I vividly remember being told a story about bees. When the story ended, we all obediently stood up to pledge our allegiance, in that col-lective monotone children adopt when reciting something they are repeating by rote as opposed to from their hearts. We each raised our right hand.

I pledge allegiance to the Flag of the United States of America, and to the Republic for which it stands, one Nation under God, indivisible, with liberty and justice for all.

Except I wasn't raising my right hand to pledge. I was raising my hand because I needed to pee. Urgently. I was waving, trying to get someone's attention. The teacher saw what I was doing and subtly cocked her own raised hand, warning me to stop. Wait. Pipe down. But I couldn't. Slowly at first, and then in a rush, a stream of warm liquid ran down my legs, on to my little white ankle socks and lace-up shoes. I froze.

Assembly finished, we all filed out, heading back to our classrooms. The four children behind me circled the puddle I'd left, and giggled. My first walk of shame, aged five.

As we reached the door, a teacher bent down to talk to me. 'Come with me to my office, Sarah,' she instructed.

I squelched obediently across the courtyard behind her. She opened a drawer in her desk and pulled out a pair of pants. They had blue dots on them. When I'd changed out of my own, she put mine in a see-through plastic bag and neatly tied a knot in it. She stickered it with a label and wrote 'Sarah Forbes' on it in red pen. Like forensic evidence.

'I will put this on your peg, so you can take it home to your mom this afternoon,' she said.

At going home time I stuffed it into my lunch box, alongside the crusts from my tuna sandwich and a half-gnawed carrot. My socks were dry and crispy. On the bus, I took out the bag and stuffed it under the seat.

I told my mum what had happened, the second she picked me up from the bus, reliving the raw humiliation and embarrassment, fat tears plopping down my cheeks. She wiped them away with a Kleenex that smelt of lipstick and Juicy Fruit gum.

That evening, I met my future husband.

Johnnie had a part in my dad's film. Just as *King Rat* was my dad's breakthrough Hollywood film, this was Johnnie's first sojourn to America as an actor.

My parents used to throw informal supper parties at the weekends and invite the cast. George Segal, James Fox, Denholm Elliott and John Standing would roll up our steep drive in open-topped rental cars, and I would hear the music from their radios die as they turned their ignitions off.

On this occasion, I was waiting. I was allowed to stay up past my bedtime as a 'special treat' and hand round nuts and crisps to the guests. I remember them all being nut brown and skinny (the film was set in a Second World War Japanese prisoner of war camp) and the balmy evenings would be full of laughter and spiralling cigarette smoke. Johnnie belonged to that small group of grown-ups who bothered to actually talk to a child without patronising them. He wanted to get the results of the baseball game, and I offered to show him my very own television set in my bedroom.

'I'm sure Johnnie doesn't need to see your TV, darling,' laughed my mother as she gathered me up for bed.

But he did. Or he feigned some serious interest in seeing it, and even acted surprised when I showed him how I could switch it on by myself. He was transfixed by my television. It was the first time in his life he'd watched a programme in colour. And that just about summed up our early friendship: mutual admiration. He admired the fact I had a colour telly, I was puffed up with the fact he was watching it at the foot of my bed, thus stretching my bedtime out by a full five minutes.

When his wife, Jill, joined him on location some weeks later, they offered to take me to Marineland on an outing. Marineland was billed as the largest oceanarium in the world, full of killer whales, performing dolphins, sea lions and sharks; home to two orcas called Orky and Corky. I guess the Standings would have felt slightly foolish going without a child, and I was thrilled at being allowed to go with them.

It was such a red-letter day in my calendar, my father took two Polaroids of the occasion. Polaroids were pure magic. In those days they had to be shoved down the front of your trousers and warmed up against your groin whilst they developed. Sometimes they didn't, and there'd be a Jackson Pollock-like stain of leaked chemicals bleeding across the shiny paper, but most times the big reveal was a good one. Faded faces gradually deepening and becoming defined.

We are posing by Johnnie's Mustang parked in our driveway. I'm grinning wildly, my hair held back by a wide headband, wearing an outfit which today would be deemed provocative and inappropriate. A short, very short, sassy dress typical of the type children wore in the sixties. It was white, and I am clutching a minuscule plastic handbag I apparently insisted on bringing. Johnnie has one arm outstretched on the bonnet of his car, squinting in the sunlight. He's shirtless and his chest is throbbing with youthful muscle definition. Great core.

The Polaroids have miraculously survived. I peeled them out of a family album when my father died. Faded a bit with age, but a historic moment frozen in time. I still worship handbags, and Johnnie still loves TV. So perhaps it's not surprising we were destined to meet again and get married, nineteen years later. I still remember our first ever date.

Weirdly, that handbag is one of the few items I still own that has survived my childhood. It was a happy day.

Today, however, is not a good day. I've woken up feeling murderous and gagging to hold my own pity party. I lie in bed and feel totally disenfranchised. It's as though my old life – my old body, my old existence – is a foreign country that I am drifting away from. I've lost my passport and all the visas that were stamped within. I'm blank. I'm devoid of optimism, and a positive attitude eludes me. I've got so few eyelashes left, even a pinprick of tears gushes straight down my cheeks; they no longer get caught. There's no barrier to hold my emotions at bay.

I pick a fight with my mother on the phone for no reason. I tell her I'm going stir crazy. I haven't sat down indoors and talked face to face, at close quarters, with anyone other than my husband and masked hospital staff, since the beginning of November. I'm held hostage within my house. Yes, we are all in lockdown round three, but for me it feels as though I'm rolling two dice. And scoring two sixes. I'm both in Covid lockdown and cancer lockdown. Hell. Whatever anyone says, whatever well-intentioned rhetoric is spouted about how we are 'all in this together', I don't feel we are. I feel excluded. Blackballed.

I can't find it in me to feel grateful for anything today. Not for the clear blue sky. Not for the nice lunch a neighbour has dropped off. Not for the fact I have walked with Johnnie to a new bread shop down the road and waited, masked, like a leper, keeping my distance across the road, whilst he went in and bought me a cheese roll and a cup of coffee. I wanted to be in that shop. I longed for a basic exchange with a stranger. Pathetic goals, but nevertheless real to me.

I don't think my mother understands why I am angry. I'm angry because she always tries to talk me down from an emotion that I own, instead of just accepting the fact it exists. Or else she equates it back to herself. She compares and contrasts, telling me she too feels lonely and isolated. And instead of making me feel better, it just makes me feel guilty, cross and helpless. Because I can't do more for her.

I can't always look on the positive side and project forward to March, when I will have finished treatment. A big part of me thinks cancer never ends for the person who has had it. It's not a fairy tale with a happy ending. It's a Grimm's forest that can become scary at any given moment. The safety net of good health has been whipped away, and never again will I be able to dismiss a weird twinge or ache, nor treat it with indifference. I will forever be a nightwatchman, searching for signs my luck has run out. My torch always casting its light on the lurking shadows. Fuck you, cancer, for ruining my sunny disposition. I will never forgive you for that.

Just as being urged to think of all the starving children in far-off places failed to encourage me to eat all my broccoli as a child, so too does comparing my current situation to everyone else's fail to resonate with me and improve my mood. I'm too curmudgeonly. Too self-centred and selfish. Today I just want something I very seldom ask for: I want sympathy. Like I said, the invite to the pity party – a personalised invite for one – is up on my mantelpiece today. I've ticked to say I'm attending.

So far, I've managed not to leave my calling card with Mr Sympathy. I haven't demanded it, nor have I sought it. I genuinely just want distraction; something to while away the hours. But time is moving like treacle, and I am like a bulimic needing to binge on any outside news I can lay my hands on.

Lockdown isn't bringing Covid numbers down; they are skyrocketing. Terrifying. And then Tilly tests positive. Far away from home. My daughter Tilly. My maternal umbilical cord severed by rules. I can't take care of her, for the first time in both our lives, just as my mum can't take care of me. I understand the agonising wrench.

Felix is taking care of her. I listen to her little, weakened voice on the end of the telephone, reassuring me she will be okay, telling me she just feels very, very tired and has a horrible headache. Johnnie is deranged with worry and helplessness. I realise, with a thud, I have no choice but to park my fears.

I can't do what every fibre of my body is programmed to do: I can't mother her. I can't rush out and buy nourishing soups and juices, and more paracetamol, and a bunch of flowers, and make a cauliflower cheese to stick in the oven for supper. I can't make her bed comfy and see with my own eyes that she hasn't got rapid breathing or Covid tongue, Covid toes or a temperature. We are totally isolated from each other.

This is the real cruelty of being ill today. We have to face it all alone.

12

I go back to hospital – alone, again – for my fourth round of chemo and yet another PET scan. I have to fast prior to the scan, so I arrive feeling empty, hungry, decaffeinated, weak, full of water and dizzy. In my bag, a little square of banana bread wrapped in tinfoil sits waiting to be popped into my mouth the second I emerge from the machine, my veins pumping with injected radioactive chemicals that turn my pee fiery hot and red.

The subterranean hospital rooms where all the MRI, CAT and PET scans are conducted are strange, silent places. They remind me of experimental labs or sets from a science fiction movie. The patient is positioned precisely and then left while the technician operates the machinery from behind a glass window. These vast, futuristic, predatory beasts allow no hiding place for secrets. My body may be partially clothed, but make no mistake, this is a diagnostic rape. Full exposure. Every shadow, every tumour, every cancerous spot, every growth is illuminated, marked, revealed.

'Music?' asks Alan, as he covers me in a blanket and asks me to position my hands above my head.

'What are my options?' I ask.

'I can only get romantic classical,' he replies.

'Fine.'

Out drifts the theme song from *Doctor Zhivago*. The haunting sadness of Lara's tune when she leaves Yuri.

I remember seeing that film for the first time at the Paris Pullman, a little art house movie theatre just off the Fulham Road. They were holding a retrospective of David Lean's work and I went with my then boyfriend, Cassian. You could still smoke in cinemas in the seventies; the backs of seats all had little flick-up ashtrays, and if you went in the afternoons, you could happily intersperse surreptitious snogging with smoking. Legs carelessly sandwiched between the seat partitions, a packet of Poppets clasped between your knees; the chocolate always disappointingly chalky, the nuts dry.

Another romantic classical tune. This time from *Schindler's List*. The silent, all-seeing machine glides slowly backwards and forwards above my torso, and then abruptly stops.

Alan comes back in and helps me down. I get dressed and make my way up to the oncology ward. Everything has become so familiar. The corridors, the swing doors, the nurses, the room, the machinery. I am a returning patient; albeit an impatient one.

I have my routine. First, I unpack my 'chemo hospital bag'. The one Anya delivered to my room the night before I started my treatment. That night somehow seems like a lifetime ago. I was a different person back then, buoyed up by adrenaline, fear and disbelief. I now realise I was in denial. I think I'd shut down.

I had yet to fully join the cult of cancer and chemo. And it is like a cult. Truly. It's travelling to a foreign country without a passport home; belonging to a tribe that exists solely in a parallel universe. The only people who truly understand the rules are those who have already been indoctrinated. The ones who have been forced to swallow the Kool-Aid. A bit like childbirth. Once you've given birth, you look upon every mother as a potential comrade. Automatically unified by the unyielding knot of a shared experience.

Joining the cancer-chemo cult is like being christened in kindness. Overwhelming kindness. A kindness that cuts through boundaries. The tendrils creep through cracks and somehow find you. Like a raging bush fire, the flames of mortality ignite compassion. It passes with the alacrity of a steam train through the address book of your life. People you haven't spoken to for years, call you up. True friends nail their colours to your mast and just guide your leaky little boat through the storm. Cancer changes you forever, whatever the outcome. It's made me believe that innate, generous goodness is the real currency of life. The rest is just spare change.

My therapist slinks in. I always fail to recognise

Susie and assume she's a nurse come to take my blood pressure.

'Is this a good time?' she asks, as ever.

'Absolutely,' I reply, picking up the needlepoint I'm doing and threading a long piece of green wool.

'How are you feeling today?'

'Bored.'

'Bored?' repeats Susie. 'Explain your boredom.'

I put down my canvas and give her my full attention.

'Did you get away to the Maldives for Christmas?'

'No,' says Susie sadly. 'Because, if you remember, we went into tiered lockdown. I was nervous that travel restrictions would be put in place, and I wouldn't be able to return.'

'I feel much the same,' I say. 'I feel bored by restrictions and cancer, and fear I may never return to normality from this unscheduled trip I'm unwillingly on.'

We stare at each other.

'Oh,' says Susie. 'I see a bit of anger seems to be edging its way to the foreground. The last time we met, I was concerned you might be experiencing denial.'

I stab the button fixed to the side of my bed and reposition myself so that I'm sitting poker straight. I'm suddenly sullen. I'm sullen in the same way a teenager is when receiving a bollocking; staring ahead, buying time whilst desperately thinking up an exit strategy.

'I'm not in denial, Susie. Who comes into hospital every three weeks, with a Portacath semi-permanently fitted beneath their breastbone, wearing a beanie because they are totally bald, has a mouth that feels as though it has licked a car engine, numb toes, a withered body, aches everywhere, and hangs about talking to a therapist whilst a cocktail of toxic drugs is being prepared to pump into their body? How can I possibly deny I have cancer? I'd have to be either a masochist or a moron.'

I'm on a vicious roll now. 'Obviously, I want to break free. I would be a freak if I thought otherwise. I dream of breaking free, just like you dream of jetting off to blue seas and warm sands. It's not just the Maldives that have been put on hold for me, Susie. It's my entire fucking life. And I'm bored. Bored at how much my life has shrunk. Bored by the boringness of not seeing anyone. Bored by the monotony of my days. Already bored by the boringness of the days I know I still have ahead of me. I'm bored by people telling me I'm halfway through, bored of waiting until March. But most of all, I'm bored of myself . . .' I pause. 'Because I am bloody boring. I'm a bore. I feel it, I know it, and I am it.'

I finish my monologue. I have a feeling I'm presenting a bit of a challenge to poor old Susie.

'Okay. Try and project yourself forward to the end of your treatment,' she suggests gently.

'Will do,' I reply.

And that's that. I'm saved by the next chemo concoction bag arriving.

Today there is a young student nurse shadowing Gary. Gary is great. It always amuses him that I screw my eyes tight shut while he activates my port and attaches the gripper.

'What are you like?' he says. 'What the eye doesn't see, the heart doesn't grieve over? Is that where you're coming from?'

'You've got it, Gary,' I say, laughing. 'Is it done yet?'

'All done. Fit to be seen. Now, Mia, have you dealt with a port before?'

Mia has to endure something insane like 2,000 hours of unpaid practical work before she completes her training and qualifies. Make no mistake, nursing is a selfless vocation. Today she is Gary's bitch, rushing off to find some gauze, a tube, a Band-Aid. Wheeling in the blood pressure machine, clearing up and disposing of the endless detritus created whilst flushing out my various lines.

Gary sits close as he administers the three huge Red Devil cocktails by hand; pushing the plunger slowly into the gripper attached to my chest. I feel the strange menopausal headrush of heat boil me momentarily. It's familiar now. I no longer wonder what's happening. I know what's coming.

Dr Plowman rushes in.

'Was my scan okay?' I ask, immediately cutting to the chase. 'How's the tumour looking?'

'Progressing nicely,' he replies, looking down at his notes.

I've heard it before. I'm gutted. Floored. Nonplussed. It sounds a bit like a school report. Nice is such a non-event. Nice is never what one wants. Nice boys are boring. Nice tasting is dull. Nice looking is seldom very handsome. A tumour that is 'progressing nicely' needs to get a grip, buck up, hurry up and fuck off forever.

Not be nicely progressing.

The party is over. The post-chemo steroids no longer give me the insane, adrenaline-charged, five-day high they did at the beginning. The false sense of security. When they worked, they used to make me feel invincible. The medicinal energy they pumped through my system obviously overrode the crushing effects of chemo running wild throughout my body. They made me feel strong and reckless. They were my saviour.

Steroids are strange drugs, and bizarrely I miss the effect they used to have on me. Firstly, I'd put on nearly half a stone in weight, immediately. Overnight. Like being inflated by a balloon pump. My face became rounder, and I'd develop a little pot belly. They made me insanely thirsty. The sort of thirst normally associated with being hung-over. I guzzled water so fast it would drip down my chin. I felt hungry. A nasty hunger unconnected to my head; the type that stabbed at my stomach lining, like certain strong antibiotics. A persistent demand to shovel food down in order to silence the growl. All these symptoms were not nearly as unpleasant as they sound, because, ultimately, they made me feel oddly alive. On edge. After five days, everything reverted to normal. Well – a new normal. The gained weight disappeared overnight, the cheekbones returned, the hunger abated, the faux energy levels levelled out.

I've become used to the caterpillar-to-butterfly cycle. But this time it hasn't performed its magic. I'm a slug.

I feel lethargic. Slow. Unmotivated. Slightly removed from the action, as though my voice and thoughts are muffled. It's like swimming underwater when you hug the bottom of the pool, aware of the milky, filtered sunshine above the surface but unable to feel its heat. I feel sad. And I'm not used to feeling sad. I've joined the underbelly of cancer; and I feel I'm vulnerable to attack. And no one can take that feeling away, least of all me.

I spend a lot of time just thinking. Doing nothing, just flicking through the Rolodex of my mind, remembering the strangest things. The little 'freeze-frame' moments of my life. The more inconsequential and smaller my everyday routine becomes, the more my memory collates fragments from my past. It's as though I'm making a personal scrapbook, in case I'm not around one day. Reminding myself of the good times I've had. And they are never what you imagine they'd be. They are just everyday life.

I remember being about four years old. I can see myself lying in my bed beneath a hot sheet. My embroidered nightie rucked up around my thighs, thumb in mouth, teddy bear clasped to my chest. Summer bedtimes always seemed so unfair when it was still daytime outside. The humid air buzzing with midges, a bird's cry in the far distance; echoes of adventures hanging in the ether. The curtains failed to promote the impending nightfall; they just billowed and teased, wafting the early-evening heat around my room.

I kept ladybirds by my bed. In glass jars that I'd turn into elaborate terrariums. I'd collect specimens from the vegetable garden; searching through the runner beans that grew up bamboo canes, tied together like wigwams, and ferreting about the raspberry bushes. It required a certain skill, and I had my fair share of injuries. I was fascinated by ladybirds. Their deep orange colour, their spots, the way they produced foamy lava. I felt a strong moral obligation to rescue them and not let them be homeless.

> Ladybird, ladybird, fly away home!
> Your house is on fire, your children all gone;
> All except one, and that's little Ann,
> And she has crept under the warming pan.

As long as they were next to my bed, nestled in a screw-top jar with air holes punched into the lid, I reasoned they were safe. I always made sure they had a couple of leaves, a twig or two and a splash of water. But as I checked on my charges this particular balmy night, I could see they'd died. I'd failed them. They were balled up and crunchy, the leaves had started to turn to dust, and their already fossilised corpses were just rolling about like miniature marbles. I was devastated.

I ran downstairs, clutching my jar like an urn full of beloved ashes, and found my parents sitting outside on the terrace. I was sobbing. My heart was broken.

'We will find more,' announced my father.

And the three of us held hands and walked across the crispy grass, heading towards my old hunting ground. My bare feet tippy-toeing in order to avoid treading on the razor-sharp, spiny seed balls that hide on lawns.

We found a lone ladybird, curled up ready for the night, and plopped it into my jar, where it rolled around with the corpses.

I was tucked back into bed, the pads of my feet blackened by earth, and I stared at the jar until dusk hit, darkening the room.

And then there were my chickens, the naming of which coincided with my short-lived religious period. Jesus and Nazareth were two struttingly proud hens who lived in a coop at the end of the garden. I loved them, and was completely undaunted by their bony bodies, beady eyes and gelatinous feet.

I talked to them and poked bits of grass and squishy apples through the wire mesh, before surreptitiously sliding open their cage, blocking their escape with my determined little body. Once inside, I would dive into their enclosed nesting area, oblivious to the squelch of green runny poos. I would inhale the smell of straw, and ferret about for eggs, pushing the chickens away if they attempted to get too territorial.

'Move over, Jesus,' I'd say bossily; my lisp probably fudging the pronunciation.

My Sweet Lord would get all flappy and throw himself against his cage, but I didn't care. I'd put the foraged egg in my duffle coat pocket and sit happily in the mud, having long conversations with my feathered friends. And then one day I upped the ante. I asked Jesus to give me a baby sister. I was deadly serious and did so with no doubt in my mind whatsoever that my prayers would be answered.

And hallelujah! The following year, Emma was born, and I callously gave up both my obsession with chickens and my religion. I had a real chick to boss about and love.

My new obsession at the moment is being vaccinated against Covid. I believe wholeheartedly in vaccinations. I've grown up with them and can vividly remember being given a white sugar cube to protect against polio as a small child. I vaccinated all my children, against everything I could. I never agonised over the pros and cons.

It's the same with my treatment for cancer: I trust the science. Whilst I'm touched by offers to 'heal me through music', or suggestions that I switch to a Keto diet, alternative medicine, and forgo the chemo, I'm welded to a system that builds and organises knowledge in the form of testable explanations and conclusions. And as far as I'm concerned, science is the driving force that projects us forwards. I want to be vaccinated against Covid-19 – I want everyone to be vaccinated – because not only do I believe it is the only way out of this pandemic, I also believe we all have a moral duty not to opt out. We can't be selfish on this one. This virus is too explosive to just blithely walk around acting as a potential hit man.

I want to go back to trusting. I hate the way I compartmentalise people and mentally label them 'safe' or 'rogue'. I avoid the rogues like the plague. I cross the street, step back, avoid at all costs. I don't want to live like that. I don't enjoy being judgemental.

So I become a pest. I pester the hospital, my doctors, my oncologist, with the tenacity of a pit bull. I'm jealous when Johnnie, because of his age, qualifies to receive the Pfizer jab, and I'm ecstatic when he receives his second one. One small step towards freedom.

When I first became ill, the general consensus was that I would have to wait until I finish treatment to be inoculated. But now, as is often the case with science, the goalposts change. It seems I will qualify, but only if I can get it a week after I've completed a chemo cycle.

Except. Except. Except the only time it is happening in my area is on day five, not day seven.

'Mmmm, not ideal,' says Dr Plowman. 'But I think it probably would be prudent if you seized the opportunity.'

Saturday morning, and I virtually skip to the vaccine centre, roll up my sleeve and truly savour the experience. So beautifully and safely organised. It makes me proud to be British, and I leave feeling I am inching closer to leaving purgatory. I can see the light at the end of the tunnel. The freedom pass is swilling around my system, and it is like being infused with optimism.

I don't feel quite so optimistic the following morning, however. I'm not sure if I am suffering from the fallout of the vaccine clashing with chemo, but all I know is I

192

wake up with every vestige of energy sucked out of me. It is as if I am standing in the eye of a Covid-chemo cyclone, trying to keep upright in the wind. My body feels boneless, and I barely have the oomph left in me to talk.

Strangely, cancer has never made me feel clinically ill. I don't know if this is because of the type of cancer I have, or the way my body has responded to treatment, or simply the fact that I've had the formidable (Red) Devil on side, but I've somehow avoided feeling properly ill.

And yet I don't feel normal any more. I walk around all day experiencing acute, out-of-body sensations I struggle to take control of. If I bend down, I feel faint. If I get up too quickly, I can feel my sap rising like mercury in a thermometer. I get massive headrushes like tidal waves. I feel them climb, then stay static for a few seconds, and I just wait patiently for the thunderous crash I know will follow. The tips of my fingers are numb, and my phone no longer recognises their imprint. My feet have no feeling. They are dead.

I never used to think twice about being alive, whereas these days I must try bloody hard not to focus on all the signals my body is sending me. Up until now I've never needed to consult the manual. Everything about me just worked. Effortlessly. Cancer has changed that. I'm inhabiting a body that obviously belongs to me, but I have no notion how to make it function. It has a new set of rules.

It's like dealing with one of those highly complicated Lego instruction leaflets. All the right pieces are spread before me, and I've just about managed to build the base, but I'm buggered if I can make the main tower stay on securely. It wobbles. Like me.

I think I'm suffering from depersonalisation. A detachment of self.

It's a genuine thing; I feel like a removed observer of myself. I fear I have changed irrevocably. The world has become almost dreamlike and I am outside reality, looking in.

I don't know who I am any more.

13

I looked at myself in a full-length mirror yesterday and was appalled. Naked, I looked exactly like one of those anatomy posters from the fifties. Not the one that revealed a cross-section of the body's internal organs, but the one that showed veins, sinews, muscles. I stood in the same position as the figure in the drawing; legs slightly akimbo, hands in a downward welcome gesture, bald head looking straight ahead. The damage is strangely mesmeric.

For starters, my body seems to have become transparent. I can physically see the pathways of my blood vessels beneath my skin. They resemble one of those complicated colouring pages grown-ups like to fill in, to help beat stress. Repetitive patterns. I have flesh on my arms but it has lost its grip on my muscles. It's almost a pre-pubescent body in some aspects. It has a silky, hairless smoothness to it. My breasts are like little afterthoughts. And my head. Rounded with baldness. Alien to me. My forehead larger and more looming than I was aware of when it was covered with hair. Two tiny but prominent veins at my temple.

My face is undeniably tanned compared to the rest of me, and I imagine this is due to some odd chemical legacy caused by chemo. I still have eyebrows, albeit sparse ones, for which I am extremely grateful, but my eyelashes are pathetic. Lack of eyelashes makes my eyes seem both staring and dull.

I am totally detached from this person. I feel as though I'm waiting to get dressed in a bodysuit that's hanging in my wardrobe next door. It's hard to describe how strange it is to look like someone else when I've lived with myself and all my imperfections for sixty-one years.

I want to walk away from the imposter. But I can't.

Instead, day after day, I have to invite this weirdo into my life. Welcome her. I have to use reverse psychology. I put on a costume and get made-up in an attempt to disguise her and morph back to being myself again.

I don't wear tight clothes, although it's tempting. That would draw too much attention to the withering. I layer up. I wear make-up. Every day. I darken my eyebrows with a spindly little brown stick. I gently apply mascara to my pathetic lashes; and a carefully applied thin line of kohl to my outer eyes. I put on concealer to cover up my dark circles. I use a subtle blusher. I oil my skull with coconut oil and massage it in. And when I've done all this, and look at myself under a harsh light, before I've put on a fresh beanie or my wig, I look exactly like a drag queen. A performer waiting to inhabit a role.

Lights. Camera. Action.

Put on a happy face. Roll up. Roll up. Let the show begin.

As Frank Ebb says, 'Life is a cabaret, old chum.'

It's strangely cathartic if I imagine I am playing a part; if I fantasise that I've left the real Sarah Standing sitting in the audience whilst cancer victim Sarah, made up and in costume, is just a fictional character. I'm a method actress. I know my lines. But what keeps me sane, and what keeps me going, is the act of telling myself this production of mine will eventually end. The show will close. And one day, I will get to walk away from this intense role I've been inhabiting for the last three months.

I will step out of the limelight, leave the stage, close my dressing-room door, hand the key back to the stage doorman, and revive a part I've played before.

Myself.

I was very much myself when I attended my local village junior school. Pigtailed, wearing a grey tunic and red ribbed socks, sitting at a splintered wooden desk in a dusty classroom. The air permanently speckled with particles of chalk. Teachers who seemed older than God. And no mod cons. How different schools were, back in the days before Health and Safety kicked the shit out of the curriculum. We sang exclusively Christian hymns at assembly, were given mini cartons of milk at break, together with a malt biscuit, were allowed to climb trees unsupervised at break, and had a proper uniformed matron who didn't have to seek parental permission to dole out Junior Aspirin.

In fact, parents were pretty uninvolved with their offspring's schooling, pitching up only at going home time and the annual Christmas concert.

I loved it. I loved my exercise books with their Farrow & Ball muted covers: green for sums and times tables; pink for writing and stories; blue for history; grey for geography. I loved the daily nature walks through the overgrown field that backed on to the playground, searching for stick insects and butterflies, picking buttercups and daisies to press between sheets of pink blotting paper, and collecting leaves.

I loved lunch. Sitting at long, narrow tables with a teacher at the head doling out fatty slices of lamb, watery gravy and overcooked vegetables. I especially loved Thursdays, when we got steamed treacle pudding and custard with a skin on it that was congealed and almost impenetrable. I hated Tuesdays, when it was rubbery, acrid-smelling liver (which always seemed to have green veins) followed by tapioca pudding with bowls of strawberry jam with bits in it. I would chew the liver, over and over, before coughing it into my fist and dumping it beneath my feet, where I would grind it into the green linoleum with my Clarks shoes. I still hate it to this day.

What I liked most was what happened after lunch. We would line up, vying to sneakily position ourselves next to our best friend, and troop into what was grandly known as 'the Library'. Another schoolroom with wide, worn wooden floorboards and free-standing bookshelves packed with higgledy-piggledy books. We would each grab a cushion from a stack in the corner, and prepare to listen to the BBC Home Service on the radio.

As the milky sunlight filtered through the large windows and made patterns on the ceiling, I would lie, sucking my thumb, and go into a state of complete entrancement. Listening to the clipped tones of an educational broadcaster transporting my imagination to another world, another country.

I remember a girl called Margaret, from the form above, who once sat up in the middle of rest time and was violently sick. Funny, the things that are forever stored on one's memory stick. The teacher quickly took her up to Matron. We all got up as soon as she left the room and gathered round the pool of chunky, putrid vomit, staring at it in fascination. We got into big trouble when the teacher returned with a red bucket of sawdust. She threw it officiously over Margaret's mishap, before another teacher arrived with a dustpan and brush, a bucket of hot water, disinfectant and a smelly mop.

Gym every day was considered important, and I wasn't very good at it. A lot of balancing on narrow raised benches, skipping, vaulting, relay races with bean bags, and doing running jumps over sticks of bamboo held up unevenly by two volunteers. The ignominy of being one of the last to be chosen for a team.

I don't think we ever had homework. We'd just have our Peter and Jane reading books in our satchels, and endless 'artwork' stinking of cat food. That's what Copy-dex smelt like, and we would use it liberally to stick on bits of tissue paper, creating a collage.

At the end of the school day, it was home to another biscuit break, then supper and *Blue Peter* before bath and bed.

School was simple, uncompetitive, and monotonously enjoyable.

My cancer treatment, on the other hand, is beyond monotonous and is definitely not enjoyable. It's becoming harder with each day that passes, and I am trying to analyse why. I'm on the homeward stretch, so I should feel encouraged and cautiously optimistic. But I don't. I feel gloomy and despondent.

At the start, I felt like a thoroughbred racehorse about to compete in the Grand National. I was bucking and snorting with adrenaline and fear, caged in and rearing to be released once the starting pistol was fired. I aimed to win this motherfucker of a race, and I felt I was the favourite to do so; I had all the odds on my side. I held the pace for the first lap. And the second. I jumped the fences and didn't go down.

But now, just as I'm approaching the finishing line, I'm running out of steam. I can hear the cheering from the sidelines, but it's muffled and distracting. My body, which began this race all sleek and highly tuned, is now sweaty and spent. I can feel it running out of puff. And however tightly my family, friends and support group hang on to my reins, I fear I could stumble at any moment, foaming at the mouth, crashing into barriers, riderless. I have no concrete reason to think like this. The root of my current mental state boils down to one thing: a lack of physical proof that the treatment has worked.

With a cancer that isn't physically cut out – and one I never saw or felt in the first place – I have to just believe in its existence. I also have to trust it's going away, without any tangible, visible proof. And it is hard for a realist like me to continue believing that something is working, when I can't actually see that it is. There are no weekly stats. I can't get to grips with that. PET scans that are 'progressing nicely' are ethereal.

Come to think of it, I've never formally been introduced to my tumour. Not having seen it with my own eyes on any scans, I'm left with a mirage. I mostly visualise it like a floating, amoebic jellyfish, its wavy edges undulating to the pulse of the fluids inside my body. They told me initially it was the size of a child's rugby ball, but I want to know if it's shrunk to the size of a cricket, tennis or golf ball. But they don't tell me. I've observed that doctors survive by being oblique. But I want full transparency, in order to manage my expectations.

I'm trying gently to micro-manage the expectations of those I love and who love me back. I didn't at the start; I surfed the same wave. I viewed the date my treatment will end with the same certainty as seeing a full stop at the end of a sentence. Now I see the end as a semi-colon. It's not finite in my mind. I want it to be, but it's as if I've lost my nerve.

I used to think of 7th March as the day I'd rip open the chocolate bar and find the much-anticipated Golden Ticket. All my troubles would be over. The Willy Wonka of oncologists would hand me my freedom pass.

I'd hotfoot it along the Yellow Brick Road.

The reality is going to be different. I see that now.

But this too was yesterday's state of mind. I've got myself back in the race. Somehow. With a little prod.

Anya suggests I throw off my middle-class politeness, email my oncologist and ask him for the improvement percentages shown on the before and after scans. And she's right. I need to stop being an undemanding pussy and start demanding. Like many patients, I tend to preface everything with 'I'm so sorry to bother you' or 'I apologise for taking up your time' and 'I'm sure it's nothing, but . . .' Whereas I'm not really sorry at all.

We are all allowed to wear our hearts on our sleeves nowadays. Encouraged to. Mental health matters. So I email him and ask. And get a reply.

The treatment is on course. My tumour is diminishing. Over halfway gone. Every scan is encouraging.

Everyone's state of mind is coming a bit unstrung at the moment. The war mentality that saw us obediently through the first lockdown last year prevailed, I think, because we were all so petrified of the unknown. We were like zombies.

When we were solemnly instructed to 'stay at home' by the Prime Minister, back in March 2020, although it was a peacetime order, it was unequivocal. Non-negotiable. We scurried like frightened rabbits down into our burrows.

We welcomed our confinement. Embraced it even. The sentence we'd been handed down was in order to 'rehabilitate' ourselves. If we stayed in our houses, holding our breath, disinfecting everything we touched, did exactly as we were told – didn't step out of line, didn't question authority – we might just escape our Covid-infected nemesis. At the start, unless we were the ones issuing the edicts ourselves, or manning the trenches, we were also naively confident.

We were confident the situation would be brought under control. Back then, we assumed the pandemic would have a beginning, a middle and an end. This was a moment in history. Our Armageddon. And for the generations, like myself, fortunate enough never to have lived through or fought in a war, this was our chance to prove that we too had backbones and metal. We weren't hedonistic, woke 'snowflakes' after all. We could do this. We could be obedient. We could protect others, protect the NHS and save lives, by being selfless and by sacrificing a different sort of freedom, in order ultimately to regain it.

When Lord Kitchener pointed his finger out of a

million posters in 1914 imploring 'Your Country Needs You' and rallied citizens to join the army and fight, it was an evocative war cry. Ours was different. Our poster implored us to 'Stay at Home'. It required less team spirit. We were asked to retreat into sometimes solitary confinement.

So we locked ourselves in, and spent the spring in forced hibernation. Glued to the five o'clock news conferences like coffin chasers. The scream of ambulances cutting through the eerie wastelands of deserted streets were our version of the sirens of impending air raids. A grisly reminder of the vulnerability and fragility of human lives. We were all potentially sitting in a waiting room, dreading the call-up of a cough, a temperature, lack of smell, lethargy. One false move, one terrible twist of fate, one bit of bad luck, and it could be our turn to meet our maker.

A total of 70,000 British civilians died in the Second World War, and as I write this, at the start of February 2021, Covid-19 has so far claimed over 114,000 lives. We are living through a war that deploys no tanks, no rifles, no fighter planes. Our squadrons drop no conventional bombs. Our only weapons, up until last month when the vaccine finally rolled out, were rubber gloves, flimsy masks and plastic visors.

The Covid war is an insidious one. It kills through human contact. We are all metaphorically out on the battlefield, yet our only command as foot soldiers is to retreat. Retreat. But we are not being asked to retreat from the enemy; we are implored to keep away from those we love and cherish. Children are terrified of infecting their parents; parents live in fear of not being able to take care of their children. Those who have no family fear dying alone. Each of us has within ourselves the ability to unintentionally detonate the virus and destroy our friends and family alike. It's warped.

During lockdowns it's almost as though our DNA has been rewired to go against human nature. To be safe, you must cut yourself off and distance yourself from your tribe. Don't cross the line. Shield the elderly and vulnerable, and leave them alone to fend for themselves. Give them a dark, lonely heart at a time in their lives when the sun is already starting to set. Keep children away from school and their contemporaries, just as they are learning life skills and how to be independent. Gag grandparents and deprive them of the exquisite joy that comes from being given a second chance to live out their dormant parenting skills. Distance yourself from your own grown-up children. Try to stop every fibre of your body yearning to reach out and physically touch them. Forgo seeing friends.

For this is our war. It is a war that rages within. Our world has shrunk. Where once it was our oyster, it has become a deserted beach of empty shells devoid of their pearls. The minefield that is Covid-19 requires us to retreat from the camaraderie that normally nourishes the spirit and gets us through a major crisis.

*

When we were first ordered into lockdown last year, my big fears were twofold: I dreaded anything happening to my husband and to my mother, both aged eighty-six. Both belonging to the age bracket that was being picked off by the sniper of disease. I dreaded not being able to save them.

I used to lie awake at night, haunted with fear. I would imagine worst-case scenarios. My mother living alone, not answering her phone, lying in her bed struggling to breathe, with no one to take care of her or hold her hand in her dying moments. I would project these same fears on to keeping Johnnie safe. I would fantasise about what I would do if the unthinkable happened. Would I have the bottle to keep him at home, nursing him to the best of my ability, or would I eventually be forced to call for medical help and bid my final farewell in the back of an ambulance? Unbearable imaginings.

And what if my children got seriously ill? I couldn't *not* go to them. I'd have to, even if it killed me. I couldn't *not* take care of my mother. I thought about mortality all the time. Not mine, strangely, but my family's. My own mortality, or lack of it, was something I only thought of in oblique terms. And remember, I thought of myself as lucky back then.

But it was me. It was me, goddamnit. It was me who went and got sick during a pandemic. I was supposed to be the self-appointed nurse and saviour to everyone else. I'd long cast myself as the matriarchal fixer. I was the one who was going to do a Dominic Cummings, if push came to shove. I would lie, and drive to my mother in her hour of need. I was going to keep Johnnie safe in a glass box; pumping him full of vitamin D, monitoring his oxygen levels on our little home machine, never allowing him to touch an Amazon delivery or go on a foray for food. I was going to put the fear of God into my children and constipate them into staying in their homes and resisting the temptation to ever meet a friend.

But it wasn't any of them. It was me. I turned out to be the problem. I was the one for whom the bell tolled. Oh, the irony. I have inadvertently transferred all my projected fears on to my poor family. I have handed them the heartbreak of being unable to care for me. I have bequeathed them a double dose of helplessness. They are not only terrified of asymptomatically passing on Covid-19; they are also terrified of giving me even a simple common cold. I am immunocompromised. I am the vulnerable one.

So, I haven't seen my darling mother for months, and can well imagine the maternal agony she's going through. I have seen my three children spasmodically; but only with them standing six feet away on my doorstep. I have endured a few fleeting glimpses of my grandchildren, who just don't understand why I'm no longer welcoming them with open arms, or why my hair's no longer chestnut brown, but blond and short. I have given Johnnie the unenviable task of taking care of someone who kicks against being taken care of. There's nothing I hate more than being dependent and needy, and that's what cancer has forced me to be.

However, the exact reverse is true of my friends and family. They may have kept their distance physically, but they have stalwartly remained my 'ride or dies'. Daily, I am touched by kindness. I have had to learn to accept help graciously and not feel compelled to return the many favours. To stand back and enjoy. I have had to relinquish a large degree of control, and that's been hard.

Part of my persona was wrapped up in being munificent whenever I possibly could. I loved having lots of guests sitting around my dining-room table, and always produced too much food and an abundance of wine. I liked being the friend you could rely on in a crisis, the grandmother who would scoop up a baby and embrace sleepless nights and tantrums. I enjoyed having the power to wave a magic wand whenever my kids' chips were down. Eager to take care of Hank if Archie went on holiday. I can't do much of that during lockdown whilst simultaneously trying to protect my immune system.

My circumstances have been dictated by the pandemic barrier, and I've had to create a world inhabited by just Johnnie and myself. In the theatre, without the frisson created by an audience of random strangers sitting out front, there is precious little to alter the atmosphere. I've found it's no different in life during lockdown.

A cast of two. A daily duologue with my leading man. A man I've played opposite for forty years.

Challenging for both players.

14

My dad inadvertently set me up with Johnnie. I was twenty-one and had just been dumped. I was working for a small film company as a script reader and had been given two tickets to the premiere of *Fame*. I had no one to go with and was moaning to my dad about what a loser I was, feeling sorry for myself.

'Tell you what,' he suggested. 'I happened to bump into Johnnie Standing the other day wandering down the Fulham Road. He's not with anyone and is a real gentleman. Give him a call, I'm sure he'd love to go if he's not busy. He's great company and very funny.'

I knew Johnnie vaguely. He was a friend of my parents and I'd followed his career. But not in a stalkerish way. He'd just taken a sojourn from the theatre and was starring in a massively popular television sitcom with Lorraine Chase, called *The Other 'Arf*. He was a bit of a heart-throb. Why not? I thought.

I rang, first thing the next morning. Early. It took a lot of courage.

The phone seemed to ring forever. Eventually, a voice answered that sounded like it was coming from the grave.

I immediately panicked. Lost my nerve.

'Oh gosh. I haven't woken you up, have I? I'm so, so sorry if I have.'

'Yes, but it doesn't matter. I'm awake now,' said Johnnie, clearing his throat endlessly to jolt himself back into the land of the living.

If he was surprised to be asked out by someone less than half his age and the daughter of two of his close friends, he didn't show it. He said he'd be 'delighted' to come to the premiere and would pick me up at seven.

I had a date.

In those days, I fancied myself as an edgy dresser. I owned a black vinyl – yes vinyl, not leather – pencil skirt that zipped up the back and had a chain at the hem, which rendered it slightly difficult to walk in. I'd got it at Vivienne Westwood's shop SEX on the King's Road, in 1976, just before the infamous boutique closed. I loved that skirt. I had to lie on the floor on my stomach, having smothered my torso in baby powder, in order to get into it. It was skintight. And I'm talking sausage-skin tight. I wore it with fishnet tights and a frilly white pirate shirt, inspired by the costumes the post-punk group Adam and the Ants adopted. And that's what I wore to the premiere. And Johnnie didn't bat an eyelid. This urbane, sophisticated, stylish man, twenty-five years older than I, just took my outfit on the chin.

We loved the film, loved the after-party. And he not only dropped me home, he came in. My flatmate, Felicity Dean, was still up. We opened a bottle of wine. We chatted. We laughed. I had the most fabulous evening. I wrote in my journal that night: *At last! A date with a brain.*

And the next morning, Johnnie rang me up and asked how he could get hold of Felicity.

I put down the phone and told her. I also told her Johnnie was much too old for her (we were the same age). And that he was probably trouble and, although fantastic fun, would ultimately bring her nothing but heartache. And she believed me, and I married him a year later.

I just knew he was 'the One'.

The first night I slept with him, he told me this was my obligatory affair with an older man. He was never, ever going to get married again. And as he already had one child, Alexander, he didn't feel the need to have any more children. Not at his age.

'And what if it doesn't work out?' he'd lament.

'What if it does?' I'd reply.

'I've got seven divorces within my immediate family,' he'd fret.

'I've got none,' I'd reply.

You can never accuse me of not rising to a challenge.

We got married at Fulham Register Office, having previously honeymooned in Bali, catching an overnight flight home and arriving the morning of the ceremony (a condition Johnnie insisted on, claiming that way we wouldn't have time to get nervous). I wasn't. He was.

We had three children within four and a half years. We may have a twenty-five-year age gap between us, but it works. And when people question or comment on it, I invariably reply, 'I'm the mature one in this relationship.' Which I undoubtedly am.

In marriage, especially a long one, you establish routines, customs, rituals. You have a shorthand guide to living; your unique road map, which you follow assiduously. The intricate patterns of your joint modus operandi get woven into the very fabric of your being. Embedded. The exciting voyage of discovery that takes place when you first fall in love eventually becomes a familiar daily commute. You can do the journey with your eyes closed. Knowing how someone else is going to react to any given situation is both a comfort and a bore, and you long for the unexpected boomerang to whizz through the air and stir up the monotony.

The minor hiccups of drama that take place within a long-term relationship are ultimately what keep you together. You rely on a multitude of bit players and extras to inject unexpected twists into the plot of everyday life. Unplanned encounters that allow you to ingest new information, ready to spew out and share over dinner. Kernels of knowledge and gossip that surprise your partner.

Without the benefit of outside information, you become an unwilling mind-reader. You can pretty accurately anticipate the nuance of every sentence, opinion and view your partner is likely to utter. Lockdown magnifies this ability tenfold; instead of having recurring dreams, you have recurring conversations and rows. It's Groundhog Day all over again.

Isolation is the Antichrist of marriage. It's like entering a nunnery as a serial adulterer and taking an enforced vow of silence. It's unnatural.

I never fully understood the dynamics of needing a live audience before I married an actor. An audience is their air supply; without one they are deep-sea diving without an oxygen tank. They just drown. Acting is perhaps the only career in the arts that requires other people to breathe life into it. You can't really do it solo. A musician can be penniless and unemployed, yet still play his instrument. A painter can paint, a designer can design, a writer can write: all of them can achieve results and satisfaction by working entirely alone.

When we came back from living in America, Johnnie returned to the stage and for a period of about six years worked almost continuously in the West End.

I learnt to anticipate the Five O'Clock Fear: a cocktail consisting of apathy and adrenaline. It would arrive like a mist and envelop him. He would become distracted and clock-watch. He would physically and mentally disengage from me and the children, in readiness for the night's performance. Carrying his dog-eared script in hand, like a child's love-worn security blanket, he would grab his dressing-room key and flee, making his way to whichever theatre he was performing in.

Dressing rooms are seldom glamorous. They are normally shabby, with chipped paint and a window looking out on to an alley. A narrow divan, a tiny fridge, fossilised flowers from a first night stagnating in grimy water, a big mirror and a washbasin. They are basic; like boarding-school bedrooms or seaside B&Bs.

I remember being blown away when we went backstage after seeing a dreadful revival of *Private Lives* with Elizabeth Taylor and Richard Burton at the Wilshire Theatre in Los Angeles. Their dressing room was kitted out like Marie Antoinette's boudoir. Marshmallow-thick spongey carpets, white flowers everywhere, unwrapped baskets of cookies and muffins, chilled champagne, pristine glasses. Pure Hollywood. A world away from Shaftesbury Avenue.

Johnnie had starred in *Private Lives* opposite Maggie Smith on Broadway, in 1975, to massive critical acclaim, and I wish more than anything I had seen him playing Elyot opposite Maggie's Amanda. Forty-five years later, those lucky enough to have seen the production recall it with clarity and say it was a night they will always remember. A play written by Noël Coward, two superb light-comedy actors at the top of their game, and directed by John Gielgud. Sheer quality, by all eye-witness accounts.

We witnessed a different play altogether, that night in Los Angeles. Less *Private Lives*, more *Who's Afraid of Virginia Woolf?* Real life succeeded in imitating art. The words got lost in translation. It was as though Burton and Taylor were spitting out pithy lines of regret and longing about their own relationship, and it made it impossible for the audience to suspend their disbelief. All we could see was two superstars being overly dramatic and acting out. We laughed for all the wrong reasons; knowing too much from tabloid headlines to accept the independent power of the piece being performed in front of us.

Richard Burton generously apologised, the second we were ushered into his dressing room to offer congratulations. 'It was bloody awful,' he proclaimed, with the sad confidence that comes from accepting the capricious currency of superstardom.

One of the best parts of being married to an actor is the fact you get to fall in love multiple times with multiple personalities. It's like being given a pink ticket to speed date. You get the thrill of being mentally unfaithful whilst simultaneously looking down at your wedding ring. The person you know so intimately becomes a stranger on stage, and it's undeniably intoxicating and sexy. The lights go down, the curtain goes up, and suddenly you're not with the same man you made love to last night. Nor the one who wrongly accused you of moving something on his desk that morning and annoyed you. The detritus of domesticity is left at home. I used to love slinking back into my chair and letting myself be seduced by a stranger.

I'd never attend a first night though. Too nervewracking. I'd fret.

I never wanted to distract Johnnie, and most actors perform best when they imagine they are addressing a totally anonymous audience. A blank canvas. We were so close, I worried he would pick out my laugh and lose his train of thought. If he stood centre stage and looked ahead, he might glimpse me in his eyeline, and be thrown. I'd heard his lines so many times at home, they were like strawberry birthmarks on my skin.

I'd kiss Johnnie goodbye on first nights and feel just like a parent when they drop their child off at nursery school for the first time. Sick to my stomach. And counting the hours until I could pick him up.

The nerves, for me, would arrive half an hour before the final curtain. Having waited at home, mentally running through monologues, duologues – ticking off each act and anticipating every cue – I would rush to the theatre. I would sit in his empty dressing room and listen to the last few lines spoken onstage, echoing through the tannoy system. I'd hear the pregnant pause as the heavy curtain came down. The muffled rustling, coughing and shifting of the audience as they digested what they'd just seen.

The stage manager's voice, loud and clear over the tannoy. 'Mr Standing, please take your position for the final curtain call.'

Applause.

Exhale. Relief. PHEW.

Only then did I dare to stop holding my breath and release myself from the brace position.

After the drama of first nights were over, I'd go often to see Johnnie's performance. Multiple times. I never tired of seeing my husband morph into another character. And having been brought up on film sets, I loved witnessing the fluidity and excitement that live theatre produces.

No two performances are ever the same. The energy changes. It's like walking on that wet bit of sand that lies close to the sea, seemingly smooth and even. Suddenly, it can take you by surprise, going from soft to gritty in the space of a footstep. I found the theatre like that.

Deliciously unpredictable.

Cancer is bloody unpredictable too, although delicious is not the adjective I'd partner it with. The curtain of impending drama is omnipresent, constantly threatening to drop down and interrupt the show. Cancer is slippery. Cancer is sly. It's cunning. It's the Fagin of diseases; the pickpocket that likes to try his luck the second he senses your defences are down.

There are some days when I feel I've had a clear run. I wake up without a dry, claggy mouth tasting of chemicals. I can drink an early-morning cup of tea and enjoy it. I can swallow my pills and not feel they are struggling to make their way down my throat without the aid of any spare saliva. I can have a bath and enjoy whatever scented essence I've thrown in. The overpowering floral notes of rose geranium cancelling out the stench of toxic chemo waste that seeps out of my pores, night and day. I can get out of the bath without feeling unsteady from the heat. I don't have to immediately lie down to recover from the exertion, drinking water from my bedside table in order to quench the headrush.

There are times I can get dressed all in one go, without taking a minute out to sit down and recharge my batteries. I can look at my face in the mirror and not be too taken aback by the strange little marks of discoloration that have suddenly sprung up. I can pull on a beanie or a wig, get rid of the baldness, give my wispy old eyebrows a little definition, put some colour on my cheeks, and feel I am winning.

Some days, though, old Fagin hijacks these good intentions. He appears with his cloak, creeps up behind me and, before I know it, he's robbed me of my dignity, my energy and my determination. He's taken the lot. Thief!

It's as though he's unplugged me. I feel untethered. My voice becomes smaller. It sounds reedy. The side effects of my treatment command centre stage. Instead of being content that they've been cast in a secondary role, they demand the lead. They take over, like an egomaniacal narcissist. It's all about them.

On these days, I can't escape the fact I have cancer. Nothing in my body feels familiar. My nails are brittle, yellow and ridged. They are partially discolored. Like the rings in an oak tree that determine its age, the marks on my nails bear the stamp of chemo. My feet sting and hurt all the time, despite the fact they are numb. As are my fingers. In January, I finished a piece of needlepoint for my grandson's birthday; there is no way I could even thread a needle now. The tips of my fingers are totally smooth, as though all distinguishing features have been obliterated by chemo. They've lost their dexterity.

I feel fuzzy. I have to think before I swallow because I need to muster up the moisture. I'm tired, but sleep eludes me. Days like this remind me that cancer is not a quick fix. Chemo is leaving its calling card, not just on the tumour it's getting rid of, but throughout my body. It's like a dog that feels compelled to piss against every tree trunk and doorstep just because it can.

I ask my oncologist what my 'exit plan' is. I know 'exit plan' sounds as though I'm begging to be taken to Dignitas, but on these days I can't think of a better alternative.

The best-case scenario is as follows. Last chemo session. Second vaccination. Wait two weeks. Full body scan. If that's good, then bloods taken every so often. And check-ups. Then port removed after three months. Scans for the next two years.

Worst-case scenario, apparently, would include some sessions of radiotherapy as 'a top-up'. But it's all vague.

Wait and see.

My personal exit plan is entirely non-medicinal, and weirdly mirrors the timeline just announced by Boris for easing us out of lockdown. Mine is bingeing on a Richard Curtis box set. It's seeing my family. Properly seeing them. Hugging them. Touching them. Kissing them. Holding them. They and my friends are the glue that have kept me together. They have not let me break. I haven't done any of this alone. I haven't been particularly brave, I've just done what every other cancer patient does, or tries to do. I've just kept going.

But now I'm reaching the end of treatment I feel like the character that defiantly sings the torch song from *The Greatest Showman*. I may not have allowed cancer to define me, but I can truly say it has made me into a better person. This is my new soundtrack.

This is me . . . Look out 'cause here I come.

And the new me is slowly dipping my atrophied toes back into the water. I'm tentatively regaining confidence; I'm preparing to come out of hibernation.

When I first got ill, my mind pressed the rewind button. On life. I time-travelled backwards to when I was a child. To when I felt invincible. I think it was an act of self-preservation. Rewinding took me back in time, because my past was the only safe place for me to visit. I knew the past, and my past was not only familiar; it was full of comforts.

As I get older, I find that bad memories tend to be rubbed out and all that remains clear are the imprints of high days and holidays. Snapshots of life pressed into the album of my heart like treasured souvenirs. The bad moments become a 'story' that I am able to retell, but I can tell it devoid of the acute emotions that existed at the time. The broken hearts, the failed romances, the career disappointments, the rows, the holidays where it relentlessly rained, the times when I was broke, the flooded kitchen, the sleepless nights with a newborn baby, the much-loved dog that died. These memories develop a protective barrier as the years roll by, which allows me to forge ahead and get on with living. Like looking through the wrong end of a telescope. The images are still there; but far enough away not to reveal the pitted pockmarks.

Pressing the rewind button can be a salvation when the future looks not only uncertain, but terrifying. Or so I've found. I indulged myself and regressed. Back to a time when my world was sweet, safe, controlled and ordered. Back to nursery teas and homework and believing in tooth fairies and Father Christmas. Back to a time when I could be soothed back to sleep after a nightmare, and bloodied knees could be fixed with a kiss.

I've just started to press the 'play' button and am now toying with the notion of edging my way towards 'fast forward'.

It's liberating.

I've got used to my makeover. I'm beginning to look ahead.

The crocuses are out.

Baby steps.

15

I've always been amazed by the way in which humans can change. Some live their lives like a play with no interval. Linear. They stick to the script and don't deviate. They see the whole thing through. They stay married to the same man, stick to the same job, live in the same house. Others manage to divide and compartmentalise their lives into three (or more) acts, proving that although we are creatures of habit, we have an innate ability to adapt.

The heart is hungry. It craves nourishment, which is why many people try, try and try again to feed its demands. To alter the recipe for success. To tweak it. To believe in hope over experience. They remarry. They start again. They take their finger off the 'pause' button and launch into a brand-new adventure. A new parent falls so passionately in love with their newborn baby, it's hard to imagine ever replicating the emotion again with that much intensity. Surely it's not possible? But it is, and they do. They can.

When we listen to the song of life, anything is possible.

I truly feel like these past few months will fade into a distant memory. Cancer will just be like the time I pulled the joker out of the pack of cards. I can put it back and give the deck a good old shuffle before trying my luck again. I never wanted cancer to define me, and I don't have any intention of allowing it to now.

I will move on. Start another act. Change the plot line.

This period of my life will recede; bleed out.

The cement will turn to dust.

One of the most formative acts of my life took place when I was sixteen. Having completed my O Levels at a tiny, single-sex school in Sunningdale, where I'd been a pupil since the age of eight, I crossed the Atlantic to finish my education at a vast high school in Westport, Connecticut. It was a *Sliding Doors* moment.

Although I didn't recognise it at the time, my education at Hurst Lodge in Sunningdale had been slightly patchy, very eccentric, and definitely not remotely challenging. Our headmistress, believe it or not, was the actor Leslie Howard's sister, Dorice Stainer. I'm not quite sure to this day what qualified her for the role, but she was an immaculately dressed, quite formidable woman who had a soft spot for show business 'types'. Billy Smart, Peter Finch and Jean-Paul Belmondo's daughters went there, and on Open Days we'd all try to collect autographs. Miss Stainer liked putting on ludicrously ambitious plays. We did a Pinter production once – *The*

Birthday Party – alongside a marginally more child-friendly production of *My Fair Lady*. It was fabulously mad.

The school itself was a rambling, ugly Victorian building in the suburbs, with a big garden, a couple of long, skinny prefab outhouses (grandly called the Science Lab and the Art House), a netball court which doubled up for tennis, a murky swimming pool, and a separate cottage where the Sixth Form boarders lived. Our uniform for many years was a white, sleeveless, broderie anglaise pinafore, worn over clothes which made us look like extras from *The Railway Children*.

We had compulsory daily classes in ballet, stage and tap dancing, all of which were accorded huge importance; every exam we passed was rewarded with a different-coloured chiffon scarf, tied with pride over our black leotards. I didn't have the dance gene in my DNA. It wasn't lurking; it just wasn't there. Nor did I have the body shape. And I definitely didn't have the talent. Whilst the majority of my classmates easily graduated from red chiffon to mauve, and would prance about the corridors practising their demi-plié and grand jeté during break, I remained resolutely tethered to a red scarf. I don't think I progressed much beyond barre work. And I couldn't have cared less.

I loved being taught English, literature, art, drama, Latin and French. I hated geography and was totally disinterested in all the sciences, including biology, unless the classes involved a Bunsen burner (and thus the anticipation of impending explosions) or a hapless, crimson-faced teacher struggling to teach us about reproduction whilst we sniggered behind our textbooks.

My schooldays were pure Enid Blyton and belonged to a totally bygone era. The school secretary was called Bunty. Manners were what mattered more than education. Shaking hands and curtseying, learning how to make an apple crumble and hem a skirt, singing one's heart out in assembly, and giving thanks for food before gobbling it down. It was blissful. Uncompetitive, uncomplicated, and completely impervious to the embryonic stirrings of women's rights, demands for equality and political correctness that would explode a decade later. End-of-term Speech Days consisted of cucumber sandwiches and slices of Victoria sponge eaten on the lawn, dance displays on the terrace, and silver trophies given out for good conduct and deportment.

The bar was set low for many middle-class girls in the early seventies. Secretarial schools and cookery courses beckoned, not Oxford and Cambridge; girls were placed in a holding pattern before getting married, settling down and having children. Two of my forever best friends, however, managed to break the mould and up the ante. Felicity Dean went to drama school and became a successful actress. And Sarah Ferguson married a prince.

We'd already begun auditioning ourselves with boys at the annual, much-anticipated School Dance (which took place at Wellington). We sat on the coach in a fever of excitement, dolled up in Laura Ashley frocks, applying contraband Rimmel make-up to cover our spots, smudging kohl under our eyes, and sucking Polo mints to ensure we had sweet breath for kissing. It didn't matter who you 'got off' with, so long as you ended the evening with a slow dance to 'Stairway to Heaven' and a stranger's tongue down your throat. Happy days.

I certainly knew I didn't want to go to cookery school or study Pitman shorthand. I was a stubborn, persuasive teenager who miraculously managed to convince my parents it would be a brilliant idea for me to further my education in America. Two years earlier, I'd taken a sojourn from Hurst Lodge to be home-schooled in Connecticut whilst my father directed a film called *The Stepford Wives*, which also starred my mother.

Living in a picture-perfect, New England clapboard house, complete with picket fence, I befriended a family called the Hickeys while I was there. They lived close by, in the romantically named Snowflake Lane. The Hickeys were Catholics, had seven children, a basketball hoop in their driveway, and a pool in their backyard. With so many kids, I immediately sensed that hanging out in their house was likely to be somewhat 'loose' and at the epicentre of teenage fun. And boy, were my instincts right.

Two years later, I was back and enrolled at Staples, the local high school, as a foreign student, and Marilyn and Tom Hickey agreed to house me for the year and treat me as one of their own.

Looking back, it seems unbelievable that I was allowed to do this. I was sixteen, and had led an extremely sheltered, privileged life. I'd never gone to boarding school, and had barely spent more than a weekend away from my parents.

Weirdly, I don't remember even being nervous or scared when I said goodbye to them and Emma. I was obviously sad at leaving them. But I'd left them so infrequently, I'm not convinced I really entertained the concept of homesickness. I do clearly recall, however, boarding the aeroplane to JFK Airport and being certain in the knowledge that I was about to embark on 'an awfully big adventure'.

Back in the seventies, flying itself was still an adventure. None of today's business of shuffling on to an EasyJet flight at 6 a.m., bleary eyed. You'd never contemplate travelling in sweatpants, clutching a Pret latte and a smelly tuna baguette, holding your boarding card between your teeth and bumping a wheelie case down the aisle before yanking it up into the minute overhead compartment. Back then, flying was still undeniably glamorous. It was a rarefied privilege. Special. Exciting. Getting to your destination was only a small part of the allure; you actively looked forward to the journey itself.

You dressed up in smart clothes. You shook hands with the cabin staff as you entered the plane and were physically shown to your seat. It seemed no passenger was allergic to nuts, for there were always mini bags of dry-roasted peanuts and sickly, reconstituted orange juice served before take-off. There was no continuous in-flight entertainment. There was just one communal, giant screen at the front; it would appear after lunch or dinner, causing you to crick your neck for two hours, watching whatever was shown. The air was faintly hazy with cigarette smoke, and there was often the shadow of someone lifting their baby in and out of the flimsy clip-on bassinette, which momentarily eclipsed your viewing. You were handed a Fox's Glacier Mint as the plane started its descent, to ease the pressure in your ears.

I can remember my journey to this very day. I wore a maroon denim suit from the clothes boutique Way In, and a striped shirt. *Benji* was the featured film, and I can recall almost exactly what I'd packed in my hand luggage. A strawberry-flavoured Lip Smacker, some Juicy Fruit chewing gum, a copy of the *NME*, *17* magazine, my journal, a book and my bear. The bear that had never left my side for sixteen years. My umbilical cord of familiarity; anchoring me to my childhood, yet at the same time giving me the confidence to leave my youth behind.

This bird was leaving the nest.

Living with the Hickeys was different to anything I'd experienced before. Days were very organised, with designated chores pasted up on the fridge for all the kids to follow. Washing up, setting the table for dinner, emptying the garbage, making packed lunches for the younger kids, and laundry duty.

Marilyn Hickey, mother to seven, was petite, blonde, and one of the calmest women I've ever encountered. Kind but not cuddly. The sort of woman who had to act at being cross, because it was against her innately Zen personality.

She smoked Virginia Slims and practised yoga at a time when every other woman in American was busy 'feeling the burn' and flapping their arms about doing cardio to keep fit. She had an understated social conscience; she would disappear every Wednesday, drive to nearby Stamford, and volunteer at a soup kitchen all day. She would always apply a slick of coral-coloured lipstick before her husband returned home from work.

I remember her in the kitchen, with bare feet, calmly constructing dinner every night and singing Carole King songs. Huge pots of bubbling mince that turned into something she called 'sloppy joes', served on puffy white rolls. Tuna bakes that had three ingredients: tuna, macaroni pasta and Campbell's condensed cream of mushroom soup. Chicken wings, their skins rubbed with spicy seasoning, and ribs that had been marinated in a thick sauce before being tossed on to the barbecue. On a good day, she'd mix together a Betty Crocker chocolate fudge cake for dessert, and we'd wolf it down with vanilla ice cream.

Her eldest three sons would drive her crazy when she was cooking; hungrily circling the fridge, getting in the way, and trying to score snacks. She would playfully smack their hands away, and I remember John would engulf her in a big bear hug and flirtatiously lift her off the ground. Marilyn would giggle helplessly, feet dangling, wooden spoon still in one hand. Meanwhile, John's brothers would grab packets of Lay's potato chips from the cupboard, unnoticed, and run downstairs to the den to eat them.

We girls would be on table-laying duty. Sturdy paper plates and disposable cups, big pitchers of water and decanted cartons of milk. Knives and forks resting side by side on top of napkins. A long dining table, benches either side for kids, chairs at both ends for parents.

Tom Hickey would pull up in the driveway just before six in the evening, and whichever child was dumb enough to be outside shooting basketball would be given a task the second he opened his car door. Tom had a big, commanding voice. He was an all-round big, commanding man. His greeting would invariably be, 'Jimbo, the garbage needs to be put out. Now!' Or, 'Annie, come get those bikes back into the garage.'

He needed to decompress with his martini, which he would ceremoniously mix, having first kissed his wife hello, before taking it into the lounge to enjoy before dinner. It was like a watered-down, suburban scene from *Mad Men*. He would sit in a fake leather Eames chair, light a Davidus cigar, kick off his shoes and attempt to read the *New York Times* sports section. A moment's peace. The littlest girls would climb all over him, vying for his attention and trying to grab the olive out of his drink. Tom would playfully swat them away with his newspaper, still sucking on his cigar, and entice them away from him by allowing them to switch on the 8-track and play some Neil Diamond.

I was never made to feel like an outsider or an intruder. I was included as part of the gang, immediately absorbed into their family life. I was teased, given chores, my own peg to hang my jacket on, and the pull-out bed in the upstairs den to sleep on. I felt as though I was living out a fantasy teenage existence. *The Partridge Family* meets *The Waltons* – but without the cheesy singing or being plunged into the Great Depression.

The Hickeys' house, unlike mine, was decorated in a style I would describe as pre-minimalist. I've noticed that couples who have loads of kids tend to favour sparse interiors with very little clutter. It's as if by collecting children, there is no compulsion to collect possessions as well. Lots of orange-tinged wood, floor-to-ceiling glass doors leading out on to the deck, very few paintings and photographs, and fitted comforters on all the beds, which prevented them ever looking lumpy or being made in a slovenly fashion. Girls slept upstairs on the ground floor, boys down below in the basement, leading out on to the garden and pool.

Downstairs smelt of boys' sneakers, sweat and warm Downy fabric softener; its scent constantly competing against the testosterone muskiness adolescent men pro-duce. Downstairs was louche compared to the rigorously imposed order upstairs. Upstairs was organised by Mary Poppins; downstairs by a feral escapee from *Lord of the Flies*. There was a huge room dominated by an L-shaped sofa, a telly and the litter of male chaos: clothes aban-doned on the way to take a shower, wet towels, a single sock, tennis balls, a dartboard that had fallen on the floor, half-eaten apples, and crinkled cans of empty Sprite.

The downstairs housed the laundry room. Two vast

Westinghouse top-loading washing machines, two dryers and an explosion of clothes. The clothes were simply everywhere; plastic baskets full of single socks, stacks of washed and folded sheets, mountains of blue jeans, crumpled towers of T-shirts waiting to be sorted.

This was one of my jobs: folding and sorting. I'd sit with Marilyn on the sofa next to Katie, who was my exact contemporary and soulmate, and we'd switch on some afternoon talk show and work our way through the clean clothes. No ironing. Just fold and sort. We'd have a plate of Chips Ahoy! chocolate cookies and a Dixie cup of Coke each as an incentive, and Marilyn would balance her ashtray on her knee and sip a mug of black coffee. We'd hold up each item of clothing so she could accurately identify whom it belonged to, before folding it and placing it on one of ten neat piles, to be transported upstairs on to the owner's bed. Sometimes, it took a whole afternoon to complete, and we could hear the tantalising sound of kids jumping into the pool outside. We would have to pretend not to care. Jobs were jobs. No shirking allowed. The Hickeys ran a tight ship.

They did, however, go to bed ridiculously early. The little kids were read to and tucked in, but as teenagers we were left to our own devices. Rooky error. Although we were all issued with strict curfews – everyone had to be back home by 9 p.m. sharp on Friday and Saturday nights – we inevitably found a cunning way to break free.

Tom and Marilyn had a watertight rule that as each older child came home, they would have to announce their return by barging into the parents' bedroom to show their face and say goodnight. When everyone was accounted for, the parents would turn off the light and go to sleep. Nice idea.

We'd go out the second we'd cleared the table after supper, heading out to the beach or to the local ice-cream shop, and we'd always be home by nine.

We'd troop into the parents' bedroom, say our good-nights, yawn, loudly close our own bedroom door and corridor-creep along the passage, shoes in hand, to wait in the kitchen. We'd sit, barely daring to breathe, and look at the minutes ticking by on the large clock hanging above the oven.

At 9.15 we were off, back out again, running down Snowflake Lane, ready to jump into some uber-cool sen-ior's car waiting at the bottom of the hill. And we were ready to party. Back out into the night; down to Main Beach, to smoke cigarettes, puff joints, drink warm beer, snog and boast that we'd gone all the way to second base.

We never got busted, which was a small miracle. We'd creep back home, dangling our shoes over our shoulders, dumping the sand out of the turn-ups on our Levi 501s, and all congregate in the kitchen for a debrief and a snack. Like all teenagers, we were always starving just before bedtime. Hunger driven by hormones, adrenaline, adven-ture and the delayed munchies. It was time for Eggo waffles, cooked in the toaster before smothering them in butter and syrup, swigs of orange juice, and spoonfuls of Skippy peanut butter eaten straight from the jar.

Katie always got sanctimonious watching us binge eat; for she was perpetually on the Weight Watchers programme and knew how many points were in everything. She lost the same ten pounds, again and again, and would start out eating sticks of celery and carrots, before throwing caution to the wind and joining us gluttons in the midnight feast.

High school was a dream come true for me. Staples may not have looked particularly attractive – vast municipal blocks housing various departments, surrounded by acres of playing fields – but to me it held the same intoxicating allure Dorothy Gale must have felt in *The Wizard of* Oz when the tornado plops her down into a Technicolor world. I knew with certainty I was no longer in Kansas. I knew that going to High School in America was going to change my life.

My experience of schools up until this point had been safe. Not even relatively safe; they were cushioned, protected, sheltered and safe, safe, safe. My education in England had been as unchallenging as catching tiddlers with a bendy net in a shallow rock pool. I knew how to do it. Knew the form, knew all the ropes. In comparison, going to an American high school was like trawling a vast, choppy ocean. The waters were uncharted and excitingly hazardous. The tiddlers had all been tipped out of the bucket and returned to the sea. Suddenly, I was casting my net into a melting pot of 1,800 students who represented every socio-economic group, every race, colour and creed.

This was big-game fishing, compared to what I'd been used to. It was sink or swim.

High School seniors are not wet-nursed, nannied or helicopter parented. Instead, seventeen- and eighteen-year-olds are given relative freedom and a far more democratic responsibility towards their own destiny. There is no one-size-fits-all syllabus to follow; it's more of a tailor-made timetable, intended to titillate and focus the mind. Certain core subjects can be dropped, although science, mathematics and English are mandatory, but students are encouraged to really concentrate on discovering where their passions may lie.

My loves lay irrefutably with English and literature. I was very young to be enrolled as a senior, but since the British education system was regarded as being superior, I was given special consideration for being a foreign student, and thrown in at the deep end.

Professor Leiberwitz perched on a stool during classes and used to contort his right leg, hooking it snake-like underneath the bar at the base, whilst keeping his left foot on the floor. He wore thick Peter Sellers-style glasses, beige trousers and buttoned-down, collared shirts. I thought he was old, but he was probably just shy of fifty. He closed his eyes when he talked, and transported his brilliant mind to another zone; capturing my imagination with his forensic dissections of Great American Literature. He taught his classes with the dedication and certainty of a man who held titans such as Hemingway, Melville, Fitzgerald, McCullers, Hawthorne and Mark

Twain in the same embrace as lovers. He was to words what a lepidopterist is to butterflies. And I was pinned down by his passion.

For me, being taught by him was like being given a thrice-weekly injection of literary laxative. He concentrated my mind. He released me into the wilderness and unleashed a thirst for knowledge and a water-tight certainty that I wanted to become a writer. Leiberwitz infused me with the same love of language my father had handed down to me since the day I first discovered books. It often takes just one person – someone whose opinion you value and who gives you non-parental praise – to catapult you forwards. For me, the combined experience of my imagination being held hostage by two men, both of whom I worshipped, 'had me at hello'. It gave me a determination. A purpose. An ambition. My only regret is that I wish I'd kept in touch with my mentor. I'd love to be able to thank Professor Leiberwitz; I remain forever in his debt.

I think I was popular at Staples primarily because of my accent. An English accent carried massive kudos. Teachers and students alike were seduced by it. I was nicknamed 'Limey', endlessly teased, asked if I fancied a cup of tea, called upon to read aloud in classes – 'Let Sarah read this passage of Shakespeare, so we can hear how it should be spoken' – and assailed in the cafeteria by cute boys doing bad impersonations of Dick Van Dyke in *Mary Poppins*.

I lapped it all up.

*

236

These days, I crave a far more elusive form of attention. I want to be seduced by life again.

I want face-to-face interaction with humans. With my family. With my friends. With my grandchildren. And I want it in real time, breathing the same air, in the same shared space, unmasked; and preferably in my own house.

I long for humans to space invade, to make a mess, to laugh. I want to cook big meals, for big gatherings.

God, I even long to shop at a supermarket. I'm so sick of forward planning and imagining what I might fancy eating next week and waiting to find an Ocado slot. I want to wake up and rush to Waitrose before I go to work and be spontaneously inspired. Buy a ham and cheese croissant to eat with my flat white cup of coffee. Tiny goals.

I aspire to be a desperate housewife.

I want mundane normality back.

16

We're all having to get used to the 'new normal'. I'm grabbing what I can get and am grateful for it.

Little snatched fragments that remind me of my old life are starting to flutter and stir, like ash from a bonfire swirling into the sky. I can see the sparks in the darkness. I can't quite see where they're headed, but they, like me, have left the glowing embers behind.

Two months ago, my sister launched a live Instagram chat. Already the host of a successful weekly podcast from America, called 'Life and Soul', for Emma this was initially a mere add-on. A tinkering experiment. She aimed simply to have a communal 'rant' about life during lockdown with her followers. She's far savvier than I am on social media, and having been a presenter for three decades knows how to steer an audience. What she couldn't have anticipated was how hard it is to ostensibly argue with yourself, albeit in receipt of scrolling comments, whilst juggling a time delay on your feed.

The first time I watched her on my iPhone I was in bed, on a post-chemo, steroid high. I pressed the wrong button by mistake. I meant to send a 'wave' to let her know I was tuned in, but instead found myself sharing a split screen with her. Together. Holding hands across the sea. I didn't intend to join, but I quickly realised it was infinitely easier for her to have someone else to bounce topics off and argue with, so I stayed. We chatted. We disagreed. We pontificated. We mused. We laughed. We ranted. And we raved. And when the hour was up, we were inundated with messages. So many messages, all saying essentially the same thing.

'Don't stop.'

'Do it again.'

'Can this be weekly?'

'I felt like I was having a cup of tea with my girlfriends. You made life seem a bit more normal. Please continue.'

So, continue we did, and the numbers kept on growing. We renamed it 'Rant and Rave', and for the first time in four months I had a non-medical appointment I needed to keep.

Emma and I have never collaborated on anything work-wise before, and it's joyous. We think differently, and often have strong opposing opinions that we're not afraid to put forward, yet there is a familial generosity in sharing a stage as sisters. Like lending clothes, you bask in the reflected glory of making someone you love look good. And it's given me a project. It makes me think beyond the confines of the doctors' appointments and the time frame of disease. It's another weekly marker to cross off on the makeshift calendar I've Sellotaped to my kitchen counter, because this is the first year I haven't bothered to buy one.

Week by week, we have been joined by more and more followers, from all walks of life. A lot of fellow cancer sufferers have joined, as well as nurses and lovely women at home, all wanting to be part of the conversation. 'Rant and Rave' has become my salvation. We've hooked into an army of compassionate souls hungry for a gossipy chat about what is wrong and right in the world. The messages of support I have received from total strangers who are also battling cancer during a pandemic are truly heart-warming. We DM one another during the long nights, swapping advice and tips. The kindness of people reaching out has been overwhelming.

Tilly and Felix have surprised me by announcing they are going to do a sponsored walk in my name to raise money for the charity Lymphoma Action, which Emma and I both support. They don't forewarn me; I just wake up one morning and see a photograph of them both, posted on Instagram, striding along a London pavement. Their JustGiving blurb is as follows:

> Felix and I have decided to pound the pavement for a great cause. As some of you may know, my mum got the Big C (cancer not Covid) last year, so whilst she prepares herself for the comeback tour of all comeback tours, we have decided to hit the road to celebrate her and to raise awareness for

Lymphoma. We will be walking on 7th March –
feel free to throw us a snack as we walk and donate
in the name of the Queen of Hugh Street who we
all love so much, because, you know, FUCK
CANCER.

I read it and cry. I am so touched. They are aiming to
raise £2,000 (and will end up with £10,000). It is the
messages left with the donations that reduce me to tears.
The £10 from an old schoolfriend of India's saying some
of her happiest days were spent around our kitchen table;
£5 from a student Tilly studied with at LAMDA; £50
given anonymously, from a stranger who has been following my posts on Instagram, saying my honesty has
inspired her. The unexpectedly big drops from customers who shop at my shop.

Two days after my fifth round of chemo, I receive a text
from the NHS asking me to book my second vaccination.
I can get a jab the following day. I make the appointment
and then fret that it is maybe too close to having chemo;
and I've only received my first dose of AstraZeneca four
weeks ago.

I speak to my oncologist, who passes the buck and
tells me to speak to my primary carer. 'I'm well versed in
cancer, but less so on Covid, and I'm still waiting to get
my first jab.'

It takes me a minute to realise my primary carer is
my GP.

My GP is a proper old-school doctor who started his career long before his patients acquired the ability to google their symptoms and inform him what *they* think is wrong with them. He is wise, kind, knowledgeable and measured. For forty-five years he kept a bowl of Smarties on his desk and was furious when the Health and Safety police made him get rid of them for reasons of hygiene. As an act of defiance, he keeps them in his desk drawer and produces them whenever a patient mourns their disappearance.

'Take the risk,' he advises me. 'You may feel like shit, but as you feel like shit anyway, it's a no-brainer.'

And he is right. I take the risk. And I feel like shit.

Twenty-four hours after being vaccinated, I'm febrile. Febrile in that wild, uncomprehending way small children are when they are slayed by illness. I'm time-travelling through lost hours of leaden, semi-conscious sleeps interspersed with wide-eyed, shivery sweats. My head is weighted down and I'm vaguely aware of the day turning into night. It's the same feeling I sometimes get on a transatlantic flight fuelled by a Zopiclone and two vodkas. Dribbling. Head jerking back whilst trying to tether myself to an upright pillow; sinking forwards in slow motion against the backdrop of muffled life taking place just beyond my reach.

Chemo and a dose of Covid-lite have rendered me uncaring, diffident. It's too much of an effort to stretch out, get a grip and reconnect to a semblance of normality.

I don't give up, I just give in.

*

Now it's over. The milky light of dawn filters through my blinds.

I feel like a completely different person. I've morphed. I'm no longer a limp lump of lethargy. Strange, discombobulated microseconds pull me from the confines of a watertight sleep into consciousness. It feels like doing a reverse dive. Hurtling from dark, still waters to the safe shallows where the sun spreads its warmth. Covid-lite and chemo were formally introduced last night. They shook hands and attempted to forge a friendship, but this morning they no longer seem to recognise each another.

Hallelujah! Today is a new day.

Today, I should be happy, but I've gone and done the one thing I promised myself and Dr Plowman I would never do. Idiot. I went and googled 'lymphoma'.

Big mistake.

I've sort of catfished myself by luring my mind into an extremely sick online relationship. I now know a hit man is potentially out to get me and I'm skidding from statistic to sob story, trying to find a safe place to hide. I've entered the underbelly of cancer. I've armed myself with fear. Fear of the unknown was different. I could somehow fight off that fear by mentally taking the Fifth Amendment; refusing to divulge any facts I thought might incriminate me and affect my sentence. But I've gone and blown it. I've grassed myself up.

I've bequeathed myself a legacy of facts I wish I could unsee. Too late now. I've gone on to the official NHS website, Macmillan Cancer Support, Cancer Research UK, the Mayo Clinic, as well as all the add-ons that answer such frequently asked questions as these.

'Is lymphoma cancer fatal?'

'Can this cancer be cured?'

'How long can one be expected to live with non-Hodgkin's lymphoma?'

'If it comes back, where does it normally go?'

I've not only gone down the rabbit hole, I've buried myself alive. I've entered chat rooms and read testimonies, I've looked at photographs of gnarled, horn-like fingernails fossilised by chemo, seen shiny scalps attempting to regain hair, gazed into mouths erupting with ulcers. I've stood at the gates of Hades – the underworld of health I'd kept at arm's length – and snatched it into an uneasy embrace. More fool me. What an idiot.

Scientia potentia est. What a load of Latin crap.

I learnt that phrase at school, but I've discovered there are many, many instances in life when too much knowledge is not powerful: it's just terrifying.

I never read that laminated safety card on aeroplanes. I hate flying and spend most flights in a mental 'brace, brace' position anyway, so reading handy hints on what to do if the plane plunges into the sea or catches fire mid-air is never going to quell my fears. Valium, deep breathing, Sudoku, leg-jiggling and having my childhood teddy bear in my hand luggage (to stroke for comfort) just about gets me to my destination. Just. Being given a crash course in kicking off high heels, tying up life jackets, inflating them, going down slides and releasing a whistle doesn't. If I allowed myself to fully absorb those instructions, I'd be begging for the doors to go to manual, storming the cockpit to demand the pilot show me his flying credentials, and then disembarking on the runway. I'd do a runner.

Before I got pregnant, I never listened to other women's birth stories. I figured that when my time came it would probably be in the crutch – if not the lap – of the gods. I didn't want advance warning about rips, tears, forceps, mucus plugs, meconium or emergency Caesareans. Sometimes innocence allows for sweet dreams. I'm a great believer in sweet dreams. And with childbirth it worked.

I went to Betty Parsons' breathing classes in Fulham and acted out panting on the floor and shut my eyes when she demonstrated how my cervix would have to expand from the size of a chickpea to a grapefruit. Didn't want to know. Betty told us to take Polo mints into the delivery suite, to suck during labour, and high-fibre biscuits that looked like hay mixed with Fru-Grains cereal, to ensure our 'bowels opened' post-delivery. I went to her classes twice and got bored. Figured I'd just wing it.

I was twenty-four years old when I first got pregnant. I prepared for the birth of our daughter India with a childlike insouciance. Back in the eighties, I'd only just stopped doing all-nighters at the Embassy Club and sweating my way across the dance floor to Donna Summer's disco beats, so I barely acknowledged pregnancy.

245

Never felt sick; still wore stilettoes; didn't read a single book about what to expect. I was lucky enough to have a gynaecologist who was way into his seventies and still relied on a trumpet-shaped Pinard stethoscope to listen to the baby's heartbeat. He encouraged me to drink a glass of red wine if I felt like it to relax.

I bought two flannel nighties embroidered with little ducks, knitted a truly monstrous cardigan, haemorrhaged cash on impractical vintage broderie anglaise garments from Lunn Antiques, for baby. And just kept calm and carried on. I had a tiny bump, put on 16lbs and opted for an epidural. No pain and big gain. Fuck panting.

Pregnancy. Birth. A baby. Easy peasy.

Little did I know then, but an epidural was the precursor for the cancer 'procedures' I would later subject myself to with innocent alacrity. A little prick. Nurses stroking my arm. A fucking huge needle driven into my spinal cord. A needle I couldn't see because it was all taking place covertly, behind my back. A 'whooshing' sensation of chilly liquid up my spine, and into me, and which, thirty-five years ago, basically rendered me completely numb from the breastbone downwards.

Having had the epidural, and feeling no pain whatsoever, I was calmly watching a documentary on otters with Johnnie, to pass the time, and eating egg sandwiches from M&S.

Suddenly, we heard the unmistakable voice of Peter O'Toole hurtling down the passage towards us. 'Baby, have I missed it? Am I too late? Has the stork already arrived?'

Peter and Johnnie were close friends, having worked together on two jobs. A television film called *Rogue Male*, and a stage play, *Dead Eyed Dicks*, which they'd both starred in and co-produced. I adored Peter. We'd all had dinner in Hampstead the night before I was admitted to hospital for an induced labour.

And now hey presto! Here he was.

Peter sat on the edge of my bed, lit up an untipped Gauloise cigarette, and immediately ordered himself lunch. More and more nurses kept flitting in and out, ostensibly to check up on me, but I'm certain their main mission was to catch a glimpse of Mr O'Toole; because they were all swooning with barely disguised delight.

'It might be a good idea to put that cigarette out, Mr O'Toole,' suggested one nurse timidly. 'I'm a wee bit worried about the oxygen blowing up and the ash getting on to Mrs Standing's bedspread.'

'I'll open the window,' was Peter's reply.

After about four hours, my gynaecologist arrived and suggested it might be 'more comfortable' for Peter to wait outside as I was close to delivering.

'I'm perfectly comfortable where I am, thank you,' he retorted mischievously.

Eventually, he was persuaded to leave and sit in the corridor, where he held court with an Irish sister. I could hear them both laughing as my Richter scale contractions soared.

'Now push,' instructed the midwives.

So, I pushed. Pushed some more.

'Bear down,' said my gynaecologist.

I bore down.

'Push.'

I pushed.

'Breathe.'

I breathed. I made blood vessels pop in my forehead. I pulled an ugly face. And I panted.

I now realise that may have been the first time I floated up to the ceiling and looked down on myself (not when I was given my cancer diagnosis). I saw the see-through crib, like a fish tank, waiting to be occupied in the corner of the room; I saw the dusty particles of afternoon heat dancing through the window; I saw my feet held up in stirrups and my husband holding my hand and stroking my forehead.

Time was standing still.

My gynaecologist was poised like a wicketkeeper between my legs, waiting. We were all waiting.

I panted.

I pushed.

And then I hit it for six.

And there was India. Our daughter. My baby. My firstborn.

Perfect.

Slightly bruised like a gorgeous, delicious plum. A mass of dark hair glued to her scalp; busy fingers undulating like seaweed, cupid lips pursed.

They laid her on my chest, our eyes locked and a light switch flicked in my brain. Just like that. My whole life went from darkness into light. I was a mother. Here she was. Bloodied and wrapped up in a towel. Mewing. Mine. Nothing else in the world mattered. Not the fact I was dead from the waist downwards. Nor the fact I felt as though I would probably never pee again naturally. Nothing really mattered any more, except the fact I'd made something so exquisite.

Nothing had gone wrong. She was here. India. Her name like an indelible tattoo written across my heart. I would bear her imprint for life.

Peter came back in, having spent the last hour entertaining the entire maternity ward. Mercifully, this time, he was without his cigarette. He gently picked my baby daughter up with one hand, and turned her towards his face, examining her forensically, as though he were staring into Yorick's sightless eyes.

'Hello, my lovely,' he cooed contentedly, before planting a little kiss on her forehead, then handing her back to Johnnie and leaving.

Legend.

If only I'd applied the same advice to cancer that I gave myself all those years ago about childbirth. Stuck to my guns. Avoided seeking out or listening to off-putting tales that belonged to other people.

It worked beautifully back then.

17

Getting diagnosed with cancer is the exact reverse of giving birth. Your life is eroded out of you. The light flickers constantly, reminding you of the darkness of mortality. It's everywhere; the thousand-watt bulb replaced by a candle. I am tattooed by 'the Fear'. The Fear is like a nocturnal, evil hummingbird that hovers, sucking out joy. It comes in the still of the night. Fluttering. Knocking against sweet, honeyed dreams. I try not to let it in. Truly I do. But when it decides to sweep over me, it is as powerful an emotion as giving birth and holding one's firstborn.

I pretend I'm brave. I act brave. I even practise good old Betty Parsons' breathing exercises to take control of the situation.

I play Russian roulette with myself. It's a dangerous game to play. If I don't let anyone see the chinks in my armour, if I don't vocalise them, if I don't share them, if I promise myself to just live in the day and not project forwards to tomorrow, then perhaps I stand a chance of going back to being the woman I used to be. The problem is, at 3 a.m., I get trigger happy. I pump that gun until all chambers are spent. Like Robbie Williams' sentiments in 'Feel', I'm not sure that I understand this role I've been given. I too feel like I'm talking to God and he's just laughing at my plans.

I miss out the verses banging on about not wanting to die, and not being keen on living; rationalising that Robbie was writing about a different sort of struggle. He was after lasting love. I have the love. So much love. I just don't want to ever give it up – and I've never been keener on living. 'Feel' is my lullaby, and eventually I soothe myself back to sleep.

Strange how some song lyrics can chase and capture one's mood with the tenacity of a hunter.

Today is the day of the sponsored walk. Tilly and Felix are setting off from Bethnal Green and ending up outside my front door. I feel this raddled old Queen of Hugh Street needs to seriously up her game, and I am determined to enjoy the day. They are being joined along the way by friends, family and well-wishers, and I'm going to attempt to track their progress on an app they've downloaded on to my phone. Hi-tech. I try, in my own way – in my old way – to make an effort; to provide a homespun welcoming committee. I cook. Cupcakes with smarties, cakes, biscuits in the shape of butterflies, banana bread, and a Victoria sponge smooched with strawberries and cream.

Cooking has always been my salvation. It de-stresses me. I find it extremely comforting. It's what I do. Even at the height of my withering, I was adamant I was still going to cook one meal a day. It was vitally important that I retain a vestige of normality. So now I decorate the outside of the house with helium balloons and bunting. It looks as if I'm hosting a children's tea party. Festive. Happy.

I've always loved a reason to celebrate. Any reason. It's in my DNA. I was brought up by two parents who had an innate ability to turn any small event into a grand occasion, and nothing demonstrates the differences between my upbringing and that of my husband than this showing-off gene I've inherited.

Opposites attract. By all accounts, Johnnie had an austere, quite unsentimental childhood. Because of our age gap, I never got to meet either of his parents. I only have his description, but I'm guessing he grew up in that pre-war, buttoned-up era that actively discouraged overt physical affection or any indication of wanting to wear one's heart on one's sleeve. He was taught to maintain a stiff upper lip and keep a tight lid on his feelings. Sharing was not necessarily considered to be caring. Love was something you kept wrapped up in layers and layers of paper, like an emotional game of Pass the Parcel concealing an uncertain reward. It was a private thing. The prize was there, hidden within, but there was no guarantee you were going to be the recipient. It wasn't a given. Unlike my upbringing. For me, every layer uncovered a little thoughtful, no-strings-attached gift. Affirmation that I was cherished.

When I wanted to get married, Johnnie's main objection was not our age difference, but fear of failure. Whereas it never crossed my mind that our marriage would fail. My heart was cut from cloth that drew only on optimism as a template. We were – and still are – the yin and yang of expectations. Johnnie is still slightly wary of any sort of fuss. Like many actors, he's embarrassed by up-close and personal attention. Fine, if it's deferred praise for playing a character. But with anything closer to home, he deems it vaguely vulgar and self-indulgent. Johnnie is the man who once declared it 'rude, ill mannered and demanding' to call out our private GP on a Sunday evening when he was in agony and clutching his stomach with a potential ruptured hernia. Even though that GP would have charged him through the nose for the out-of-hours visit, and would happily have treated him. But no. Johnnie would rather wait. Too attention-grabbing. Grimace and bear it. Suck it up.

I'm the reverse. If I'm given a present, such is my excitement, I virtually have to restrain myself from snatching it out of the bearer's grasp. I have to remember my manners.

Johnnie always opens his gifts slowly. Painfully slowly. He struggles to untie ribbon and peel off Sellotape neatly. He refolds the paper. He never, ever rips it. At Christmas, he waits until everyone else has gone first. Patient. He squirrels his gifts away with minimal, polite, reserved exclamations of delight. He needs time to digest joy. Invariably, two months later, he declares, 'That was possibly the greatest gift I've ever received.' Never in the moment.

I'm totally out there with my instant appreciation. In your face. I'm fairly certain I embarrass him.

High days and holidays are events I've had to seduce him into embracing. And to his lasting credit, he has. Just as I'm hard-wired to go over the top, he's hard-wired to underplay excitement. But after forty years together, he's become a really good sport, and he indulges my exuberance.

However, today we've rather reversed roles. I'm Ernie Wise to his Eric Morecambe. Johnnie's got all the energy and feel-good vibes going. Despite the cakes and the balloons and the banners, I'm resigned to being the straight punchbag and letting him get all the laughs.

It's one day before completing my last round of chemo, and I'm spent. Every reserve of energy I've managed to fire up has gone. I'm sallow skinned and having to work hard at getting sparked up. My heart is bursting with pride at the thought of Tilly and Felix completing this walk, but my body is rebelling. It's as though it realises it's about to face the final hurdle and spitefully wants to remind me to feel grateful. And I *do* feel grateful that my body has taken me this far. I just need to keep going for a little bit longer. Just a little bit. And it's hard.

Come on, Sarah. Brush the wig out, put on some foundation, draw in the eyebrows, rouge-up and paint over the fact you're running on empty. The finishing line is in sight. I change into a RIXO sequinned top, which hangs like a scratchy sack off my bony shoulders, irritating my port and reminding me that my incentive for buying it two years ago was to hide my love handles. They've long gone. I put on some high heels. I am going to act the part of Queen of Hugh Street, even if it half kills me.

I instruct Alexa to play Abba on a loop. Game on.

I track the kids on the app. Successfully.

We jump into our car and honk at them by the Embankment. We wave. I lean out of the car window and snatch a photograph to post on Instagram.

Race back home. Pump the music up even higher. Keep refreshing the app.

Now they're crossing Buckingham Palace Road. Johnnie and I stand at the top of our street with one of Tilly's oldest friends, together with her husband and baby. We all wait.

And wait . . .

And suddenly, there they are.

They've been joined by Anya and her family. Tricia. Tilly's great friend Fabian. They are all waving.

I burst into tears. I'm so happy, so proud and so touched. If they can do it, so bloody well can I.

Getting my first glimpse of them is like pulling out all the heavy stops on my memory organ. I have a vivid flashback to over twenty years ago. France. Fontainebleau.

Johnnie on location shooting Jilly Cooper's *Riders*. I'd joined him for a long weekend, leaving the children behind with my sister, which was a rarity. I was still ensconced in that tumultuous stage of motherhood and early marriage that rendered me drunk with love, coupled with acute separation anxiety. I had a hormonal compulsion to be with them all; being away from either party made me ache with longing. I was never very good at playing the 'eenie, meenie, miney, moe' elimination game. I always wanted it all. I wanted us all to be together. My maternal inner voice played havoc with me all the way to the airport. But by the time I actually checked in, I'd mercifully morphed into a love-sick wife, desperate to be reunited with her husband. Which I genuinely was.

God only knows why I'd flown into Charles de Gaulle Airport and not Paris-Orly, but there was obviously a communication cock-up. Johnnie had arranged for a car and driver to meet me. But the driver was waiting at Orly, not Charles de Gaulle. Before mobile phones, this presented a problem. I could inform neither the driver nor Johnnie that I was at another airport. Nor did I have much cash on me. *Mon français est assez mauvais.* I tend to pretend it's quite good by just agreeing with everything, which is semi-acceptable at smart European cocktail parties, but fails miserably when instructing surly taxi drivers.

Mine wasn't thrilled by the prospect of a two-hour drive. He chain-smoked untipped Gauloises and railed against the traffic. And the torrential rain. I agreed with him on both counts. And then I fell asleep. Like all mothers do, the second they are in any form of moving vehicle away from the clawing demands of small children. I woke up two hours later, and we were still on a picturesque B road, making snail tracks behind a swaying caravan. It was now raining with biblical ferocity. The taxi cab had those ineffectual windscreen wipers that pause rather than move in a continuous motion. The driver's sight lines went from clear to non-existent.

Apart from being a nervous flyer, I also hate being a passenger in a car. Especially in shitty weather. And my fear doubles when I'm in a foreign country.

The three times we've driven through India in an Ambassador taxi, with Ganesh hanging off the mirror and marigold garlands blocking half the windscreen, I've sat bolt upright in the back seat, my hands pressing firmly on our driver's shoulders. Controlling him. All Indian drivers seem to have an inbuilt compulsion to overtake, regardless of what is heading towards them. Trucks, a cluster of motorbikes, elephants, buses, camels – no matter. It's just a big, heart-stopping *Grand Theft Auto* game of chicken to them. It's a sport. Accelerate in a car that has no power and head towards whatever is happening on the other side of the road. Honk. Honk some more. And always smile as you dice with death.

'No, no, Raju. We are in no rush. No overtaking. Slowly, slowly,' I would urge, white-knuckling it and digging my nails into his back.

'Yes, yes, madam,' Raju would reply. 'No problem.

Now is a good time.' And he'd put his foot down and weave forwards at great speed.

We'd pointlessly overtake another Ambassador taxi, no doubt containing another passenger who was also white-knuckling it. So much adrenaline in order to overtake a few goats.

I did, however, want this Frenchman to overtake the bloody caravan and get a move on. I was desperate to see Johnnie.

'*Excusez-moi, Monsieur. Nous sommes arrivés maintenant?*'

My taxi driver gestured to the road ahead with both hands. Literally freewheeling.

'*Plus tard, plus tard.*'

'*Parce que, mon mari est là.*'

He didn't reply, and I caught a glimpse of the meter. It was behaving worryingly like a fruit machine. The figures were spinning and going up and up and up.

'*Monsieur, Fontainebleau est là? Oui?*'

Mr Surly inhaled deeply and swivelled his head to face me. Eyes off the road. Furious. An inch of Gauloise ash fell into my handbag at my feet.

'*Oui.*' And, patently, that was going to be his final word on the matter.

By now it was dusk. The glorious golden hour I'd anticipated raving about, didn't happen. It was just dark and rainy. I felt as if I'd been abducted; this endless journey was taking me further and further away from my children.

The taxi driver stopped. He stopped outside one of those totally unpretentious, small French hotels so lacking in exterior life it could easily be abandoned.

'*Voilà.*'

I looked out of the window towards a tiny, deserted square lined with upright linden trees. A park bench. Two street lamps giving out a diluted, lemony light, reflected in the pooling puddles.

And Johnnie. Pacing in the pissing rain. His Barbour jacket shiny and slick with water. His Trilby almost certainly ruined.

Seeing him there, waiting for me, obviously drenched with worry, was one of the seminal moments of my marriage. He may not even remember it. But to me, it was memorable. And infinitely more precious than any fine jewels or obvious declarations. It was love. Love, actually. Pure and simple. And soaking wet.

A hideous journey with a happy ending. I'd finally arrived.

Today I've finally arrived to have my last chemo session. Last journey to the hospital, my bag packed with snacks and chargers and cashmere shawls. I'm both exhausted and elated. I feel as if I've been shipwrecked for the last five months. Just floating. When I started the course, I put my lifejacket on and had total faith I'd be rescued. Some massive liner would spot my flailing arms, held high above the waves, and haul me onboard to safety. I wouldn't get hypothermia or be eaten by sharks; I'd live to tell the tale. And I did float. But I lost track of time, in the middle of nowhere. I also lost track of myself.

Locked in, locked up, locked down. Both mentally and physically.

Ironically, the only time I really came up for air was to go to hospital for more treatment. Hospital was always busy. Full of people. Full of bustle. I can't think when I'm in hospital, which is a luxury. Other people take control. I give myself up, which is different from giving in. I hand in my body, and it's the only time my swirling mind gets to have a siesta. So yes, I'm exhausted, elated. And also more than a little bit sad that I'm going to be saying adios to the amazing team of people who have taken such incredible care of me.

I've bought them all inadequate presents online, and as I try to write down what these nurses mean to me, and to thank them, I realise I'm uncharacteristically bereft of words. Nothing I say seems enough. I've grown to truly love them, with their calm efficiency, dark humour and innate ability to keep calm. It's funny how one can become so attached and so reliant upon relative strangers.

I once got picked up in a coffee shop called Tootsies in the Fulham Road. Aged twenty-one, I used to go there most mornings. I'd sit on a slightly sticky leatherette seat, with my lined notebook and newly sharpened pencil, and eke out a cup of coffee for an hour or two. Trying to write. Killing time. The prospect of facing a blank page at home producing both boredom and panic. Better to go somewhere else to search for inspiration. I was truly faking it in an attempt to make it. I even went so far as to carry a rolled-up copy of the *Guardian*.

Sometimes I'd sit and surreptitiously observe a middle-aged American man who nearly always sat in the same seat by the window. He'd alternate between reading his newspaper and aimlessly staring out at the traffic. He was even-featured, slightly dishevelled and intense. Preoccupied. Oblivious to the comings and goings of other customers. He'd always leave an overly generous tip, carefully emptying his pockets of loose change. One day, he stopped at my table on his way out.

'Hi. I've watched you for a couple of weeks now and wondered if you'd ever let me draw you? My studio is close by.' No preamble. Straight out with it.

What a loser.

He wrote his name and telephone number down on my notepad, which was still predictably blank.

Bold, I thought to myself. And potentially creepy. A very, very clichéd pick-up line, and one that held zero street cred with a writer.

But I was polite. I asked if I could think about it and let him know.

He left, and I followed shortly after.

I thought nothing more about it. Until later, when I was regaling Johnnie with accounts of my early-morning escapades, in that vaguely conceited way new couples do in order to promote mini frissons in a relationship and avoid ennui.

'Who was he?' asked Johnnie.

'I don't know, some weirdo called Ron Kitaj,' I replied, full of the callowness of youth.

'Kitaj? Kitaj asked to draw you?' he asked, sounding not unlike Lady Bracknell.

'Yup. Why? Do you know him?'

'I don't know him, but of course I know of him. You must do it, darling. He's a sensational artist. Truly sensational. You'd be crazy not to. I'd do it like a shot. No question.'

And so I did.

Every Saturday morning for the next year, I'd sit – or stand – bollock naked, in Kitaj's studio. I got paid £10 an hour, and once I'd got over my initial awkwardness at being in a chair, legs akimbo, bush and tits out, tacky heater blowing, cup of coffee balanced on the floor, we'd talk. I knew nothing about him; neither his past nor his present. He knew nothing about me. But being naked made me both brave and bold. I spilt the beans and he reciprocated. He would stare at me intently before dipping his head to draw, then look up again, each time taking in every pore of my being. We talked with the alacrity and intensity of two veteran poker partners being dealt a new set of cards. We dug deep. Gloves off. No secrets. Peeling away the patina of personality; our egos stripped bare by the anonymity of an artistic transaction. The draftsman and his muse.

I feel the same way about the nurses who have taken such exquisite care of me. They are the master draftsmen – the pros – and I, their mere subject. I am clothed in their presence, yet emotionally naked. Raw. They are there for whatever vulnerabilities I can't quite bring myself to express with my family. They know I can't stand to watch my port being flushed and attached to a gripper. So whenever Bev is on duty, she always switches the TV on and cunningly engages me in some crapulous daytime talk show. They all ask about my children and my husband, and remember their names. They silently hand me a Kleenex when a tear breaks free, and one of them holds my hand every time I get a dose of the Devil. They bring me cups of tea. Not an acrid-tasting cuppa from the vending machine, but one from their kitchen. Proper tea. In a proper china cup. With a digestive biscuit. They take phials of blood as gently as they can. They weigh me without telling me if I've lost more weight. They admire my beanies or my wigs.

They are the epicentre of my tiny little world. They are all I have during treatment, and they know it. No visitors, no family, no friends allowed on this solo, Covid-ridden, spunk-bubble of an isolated journey. Just us. They dish out praise like an even-handed mother to her last child: with generosity, despite the fact they've witnessed all the small milestones a million times before. I couldn't have got through this without them.

Saying goodbye, I feel as if I'm being abandoned. Leaving behind the confines of penned-in disease and the structured routines of treatment feels both liberating and unnerving. Just as it's fantastic to finally qualify for a Freedom Bus Pass, it's also sobering to realise that the carefree dog days of summer are over, one's card forever marked.

I prepare to elbow-bump goodbye, and then Elena grins and says, 'Double-vaxxed!' and pulls me into a tight embrace.

She knows better than to crush the site of my port. Instead, she hugs me tenderly, on the other side. It is one of the best hugs of my life.

Love in a Covid climate.

18

It is all over. Done. I drive home and I can smell spring in the air. It is sunny. I am sunny. I have on a blond wig and a floaty dress, and although I am carrying my chemo bag, I am ready to put it into retirement.

Johnnie is outside on the street. Waiting for me. Pacing.

I walk into our house, but it has changed. Nothing is the same. The all-too-familiar open space containing bookshelves, blowsy sofas, needlepoint cushions, semi-hidden toy boxes stuffed with treats. The kitchen with its massive, wooden work counter and restaurant-sized oven, the scrubbed kitchen table and the little red lacquered highchair that has yet to be christened by Billy. All this has been overtaken. It is like walking into a garden that has become overgrown with weeds. Except there are no weeds: only daffodils. A duvet of yellow, everywhere I look. Fifty, sixty, eighty or more paper cups stuffed with daffodils. Trumpeting daffodils. Triumphant daffodils. On the bookshelves, tables, windowsills, coffee table – overwriting every surface with floral graffiti.

I stand at the door and just stare in wonder. It is like viewing the children's programme *Teletubbies* as a grown-up, but high on hallucinogenics. Amazing. I am wrapped in happiness. The welcome home to end all welcome homes.

Anya has planned this surprise with military precision. Apparently, as soon as I'd left home for the hospital, she arrived with boxes of blooms from Covent Garden Flower Market, and speedily redecorated my house. She's had to gently turn a hairdryer on them to ensure the buds are fully opened. The kindest, most thoughtful gesture ever.

I gulp in the sheer beauty, and it draws a line in the sand for me. Before and after. The bleak midwinter of cancelled Christmas, chemo, withering, electric heaters, baldness, numbness, disbelief, mouth ulcers, lockdown and isolation. January and February, punctuated by daily walks through treacle to a local coffee shop 900 steps away, to gain strength. Arriving, and leaning against the railings outside, masked and breathless. Pretending it was a breeze. Not daring to bend down because it would lower my blood pressure to the point where I felt faint. Waiting for Johnnie to bring me out a coffee and then snail-pacing it home and immediately kicking off my shoes and tunnelling down into my electric-blanketed bed for a sleep. Pretending I was better than I felt. Always pretending. Putting on a show. Trying to grin and bear it. Exercising mind over matter. The endless nights spent tilting at windmills in my mind, thoughts whirring frantically.

It is over. Over. I am in with a chance.

Wordsworth was right. And Anya has picked the perfect flowers to lay out before me. She instinctively knew that I've wandered lonely as a cloud. Yet she could never have guessed that I won first prize, when I was eleven years old, standing up at school assembly to recite, word perfect, this poem. For evermore I've associated it with winning.

> I wandered lonely as a cloud
> That floats on high o'er vales and hills,
> When all at once I saw a crowd,
> A host of golden daffodils;
> Beside the lake, beneath the trees,
> Fluttering and dancing in the breeze.
>
> Continuous as the stars that shine
> And twinkle on the Milky Way,
> They stretched in never-ending line
> Along the margin of a bay:
> Ten thousand saw I at a glance,
> Tossing their heads in sprightly dance.
>
> The waves beside them danced; but they
> Out-did the sparkling waves in glee.
> A poet could not be but gay,
> In such a jocund company:

I gazed – and gazed – but little thought
What wealth the show to me had brought:

For oft when on my couch I lie
In vacant or in pensive mood,
They flash upon that inward eye
Which is the bliss of solitude;
And then my heart with pleasure fills,
And dances with the daffodils.

I'm getting off the couch. I'm ready to dance with the daffodils.

But not quite. My friend Milica has died. Milica whom I've known since the day she was born. Milica whom I love. Milica who got two Stage 4 cancers. Milica who was one of the first people I called when I was unceremoniously dumped with the cancer card, alone in hospital.

'Mil, we're in this together,' I announced.

And Mil made me laugh. She always made me laugh. 'Fuck cancer,' she declared, with her deep, throaty laugh. 'Fuck it. How dare you jump on my bandwagon. You copycat. At least I got sick first and have got more cancers than you. And mine are much, much worse. You'll be fine. Thank God I've now got a partner in crime.' Ever competitive and irreverent Milica.

Even though Mil was thirteen years younger than I, and lived daily with an ever-escalating bleak prognosis, she took me under her wing and acted like a chaperone.

I was the nervous debutante, and she the reassuring voice of reason. We shared not only a dark sense of humour, but a family history. I knew every cast member within her expansive tribe. I'd grown up having Sunday lunches in her house. Suddenly, we were equals.

Logically, I guess I knew Milica wasn't destined to make old bones. I knew she was living on borrowed time. Too much spreading, too many operations, too much bad luck, too much bouncing back from the brink. But being logical was never part of our vernacular.

We would FaceTime each other before the rest of the healthy world had woken up, and long into the lonely nights when fear would fight with sleep. Propping our phones up on our knees to chew the fat, to swap remedies on 'metal mouth' caused by chemo, to compare notes on constipation, show each other the stuff that cluttered our bedside tables. And we'd laugh. Really laugh.

Towards the end, laughing would make Milica cough. And sometimes she'd cough so much she'd throw up a little bit, but she'd rise like the phoenix she was, feel marginally better, and then call back and take me on a guided tour of her wardrobe, or clear out her make-up bag and show me how to pencil in eyebrows when I lost mine. She'd make fun of the fact I'd eat healthy green soup every day for lunch, and would regale me with what crap she was ordering from Deliveroo. Chinese dumplings. Greasy burgers and fries. Pizza.

She came to my sixtieth birthday party, in May 2019, straight from the Marsden. She wore a skin-tight, purple sequinned jumpsuit and had portable chemo in her hand-bag. The girl had form. She was the very last person to leave the dance floor, her energy belying and outrunning the toxic drugs she had pumping into her veins. She had been ill for a year at that point, had taken on a lover nearly two decades her junior, and looked stunning.

I spoke to her for an hour, the night before she died. She kept rambling on because some friend of hers in America had called her to say they'd dreamt about her twice. What did I think it meant? It had freaked her out for some reason.

I told her it meant nothing. It was insignificant.

She kept going back to this dream her friend had had. She told me her body was getting weak. She couldn't keep food down. She was wrapped up in shawls and was a bit wide eyed, looking like ET. But she'd played cards with her mum and daughter earlier in the evening. And won. She told me she'd won. Winning was always import-ant to Milica.

I thought she looked a bit frailer than normal, but Mil had a habit of bouncing back. She was like the Duracell Bunny. She kept going.

It was late. We were both tired and, cushioned by sleeping pills, we said a sleepy goodnight.

'Love you, Mil. Sweet dreams.'

'Love you back, SS. Speak tomorrow.'

The next day was Mother's Day. I woke up, but my darling Mil didn't. She had won a lousy competition nei-ther of us ever wanted, nor anticipated playing. She won.

I choose to believe she just went gently into the night; finally drifting into one of those deep, dreamless sleeps that had eluded both of us for so long.

Milica wanted a huge funeral. We're talking an Eva Perón, Princess of Wales extravaganza of national mourning. Whenever we talked about death – which, inevitably, we often did – she was clear about a few things. She was greedy about it, and wildly outrageous. It became a bit like playing 'fuck or die' but with the highest possible stakes, a doomsday version. A sick fantasy game we'd indulge in, before ultimately getting bored. Mil wanted Robbie Williams to sing 'Angels'. With a full band. She wanted me to promise to name and shame and physically ban one gentleman from attending. She wanted all her girlfriends to wear T-shirts emblazoned with her self-appointed eulogy – her slogan of 'One in A Million' – and she was adamant she wanted to be buried in the same sparkly purple jumpsuit she'd squeezed herself into at my sixtieth birthday party. Because she wanted to look 'hot as hell' on her way to heaven. She actually said that.

Mil was perfectly imperfect, and she embraced it. Owned it. She loved courting controversy. Often, she'd say something just to get a reaction, and then she'd cackle loudly, diluting the recipient's shock by ending her diatribe with a theatrical 'shussh'. But most of all, more than anything else, her greatest wish was to spare her two sensational children, Jack and Sophia, from any lasting pain. She was a wonderful, selfless mother. And I loved her.

I loved her joy and I loved her lack of restraint. I loved how greedy she was with her pleasures. I loved how cancer didn't fundamentally change her. She was always reckless, and remained so. I learnt so much from her.

She was adamant, to the end, that in life you always have to metaphorically reach for the purple sparkly jumpsuit in the back of the wardrobe whenever the going gets tough.

Wear it with high heels.

Dance right up to the moment when the music dies.

Milica's funeral is tiny, because of Covid restrictions. Thirty people only. The chosen few. Arriving early outside a huge Catholic church in Soho. Standing in a holding pattern outside, like sad, masked, distanced chess players. Filing in and sitting apart, two to a pew.

We are all silenced by grief. No comforting hugs or shaking hands. No choir. All religious artefacts and the altar inexplicably covered by swathes of purple fabric. Confusing. It is because of Lent, I subsequently discover. Lent is a sombre season for Catholics. A time for penance and giving up pleasures. This tiny congregation is collectively fasting because we've all been forced to give up having Milica in our lives.

It is miserable.

I sit four feet away from her brother Cary. That is, until I am crying so much, and so is he, that we slide towards each other like magnets and break the fucking rules. It would be inhuman not to. My paper mask is sodden with tears, and I swear I can hear Milica's guttural, naughty laugh punctuated by a muted, '*Shussh*, what do you think you are doing, SS?'

She is indeed buried in her purple jumpsuit, and that gives us all some small solace. I will remember her dressed like that. Dancing at my birthday party. Alive with pleasure.

'You've got this, SS,' she used to say, with typical generosity, every time I went for chemo or a scan.

And the second I leave her funeral, I have to go off and have my final test. Oh, the timing. The irony of it being today. A scan to see if the chemo has succeeded in Chernobyling my cancer out of existence.

I am so numb with sadness, I barely notice the radioactive liquid seeping through my body as it is injected. Nor the rising heat, nor the need to do a hot pee before taking up position and gliding into the coffin-like machine.

The nurse asks if I want to listen to music.

I opt for Classic FM. Bowie's 'Space Oddity' belongs to the past.

I want calm. I want to reflect on the best bits of my friend.

19

I use the ten-day wait between the scan and the all-important meeting with my oncologist to take stock. I feel like Bridget Jones assiduously recording her foibles. Only they are less to do with romantic escapades, cigarette consumption and weight gain; more to do with loss. Actually, they are all to do with loss.

Wednesday 28th April 2021
Hair: bald, non-existent
Body hair: zero. Like a Sphynx cat
Weight: minus 19lbs
Toenails: brittle, ridged. Devoid of polish. Hideous
Teeth and gums: bad
Eyebrows and eyelashes: nil

Yet despite all the negatives, I am starting to feel whole again.

I've concluded that some people are born broken and

must work at becoming whole. Sometimes filling that gap takes up a lifetime as they attempt to Band-Aid it with drink and drugs and food and self-sabotage. They may have had parents who didn't parent properly. Lived lives that didn't cater to their personalities. Felt they weren't validated. Hated school, hated their bodies. Had to fight injustices, overcome tragedies. Lived through divorces. Been left scrabbling around in the dust, searching for a blueprint with which to forge an acceptable future. Looking for a way out.

I was born whole. I was, and am, so unbelievably fortunate. I may have been temporarily broken, later in life, but it was my body that broke me, not my circumstances. There's a big difference. A chasm of molten lava opened in front of me, but it didn't get to swallow me up. My innate 'wholeness' kept me optimistic. My past acted like a spirit level, keeping me on an even keel.

In my dreams I always go back to my childhood home; it still serves as my emotional safety deposit box. Despite the fact it was sold after my father's death (to a man who subsequently defaulted on his mortgage, causing it to be repossessed by the bank) and is no longer ours, my mind still meanders back there like a homing pigeon. Whenever I have bouts of insomnia or am worried, I force my mind to return through my old back door. Once inside, everything is as I remembered it and feels wonderfully normal.

The older I become, the more I realise normal should be reclassified as an ambitious aspiration; not something to kick against. Normal is the equivalent of reaching nirvana. Endlessly searching for the extraordinary is unsustainable – undeniably thrilling, and much needed in small doses – but normal is recognising that what we take for granted is ultimately what feeds our souls. Normality provides the building blocks to underpin our adventures. Wild escapades and hairpin turns are wonderful things to experience, but nothing beats coming home and falling straight back into the prevailing rhythms of daily life.

Everyone is seemingly happy with the results of my PET scan. But I recognise it's a mere stepping stone. It's just the start of a different chapter. The sad truth of the matter is this: all cancers are a long, unpunctuated monologue that does not allow for full stops. It's like looking up at the night sky and attempting to get your head around the impossible concept of infinity.

Naturally, I want that perfect Richard Curtis ending. And, to a degree, I get it. I have many little snatched vignettes, like the opening and closing airport credits in *Love Actually*. I can see my family, my friends. Finally. Cautiously. I can hug those grandchildren of mine. Go and spend the day with my mum. Hang out with my daughters and Archie. Maybe even go and visit my sister in California. I can move out of the shadows and into the sun. I can plan.

When I first got ill, I harboured such grand ideas about what I'd do if – no, scratch that, when – I recovered. But how quickly I've become indifferent to all the things I thought I wanted. I fantasised about fancy family holidays in the Maldives, and big adventures. I projected myself forward into an imagined new lifestyle, one that bore no resemblance to the life I'd put on hold, only to realise I already had everything I ever wanted.

I just wanted my life back. It was that simple.

The only problem is, all Richard Curtis movies are so good, so pertinent, so all-encompassing, they demand a happy ending. And of course, my story inevitably necessitates a sequel. But I don't want one. I want the end credits to roll, the music to be uplifting, and then a gradual fade out. Over. Done. I want everyone to leave the cinema happy. Sated. I want to release my kids and husband from the tyranny of having to worry about boring old me. Enough.

Because I remember, only too well, the daily phone calls to my mum when my dad was very ill and dying. Those phone calls made my heart stop. I never turned my phone off. I was always deeply concerned about them both. But looking back, I'm ashamed to admit I had selfish thoughts. Sometimes I wanted to get the pink ticket – just a day pass – to get on with my own life. I wanted to hear Mum say that Dad was okay. That he was okay for today. Phew. A mini reprieve. Because I wanted to get on with my own relatively carefree living for another day.

How awful is that? What a terrible admission. Why does the pounding thrust of life drive us to feel like that?

What made me so self-absorbed that I was willing to

compartmentalise aspects of my life and rank my parents lower in generational importance? My urge to live is greater than yours, therefore tell me today is a good day and I can get on with living. How could I?

I loved my dad passionately, yet I was willing (and at times able) to put his life in a box. Purely because there were times when I wanted to concentrate on my own life. I wanted to live it to the full, without shadows creeping in. Enjoying my husband. My kids. And yet. And yet . . . I would be drawn like the tide to drive down and see my dad. Often. Twice a week. If there was a crisis, I'd drop everything. Cancel everything. Skip work. I'd race down the motorway, impatient at any minor delays.

I'd lie on his bed and stroke his hand. I'd try to engage him in news. I'd read him an article from the *Telegraph*. Or the *Spectator*. For that used to be our thing. Sharing everything. Words. Arguing. Agreeing. But he lost interest. As life – his life – faded, he ceased to care. The words blurred. He stopped really listening. And I was left trying to engage my giant of a father, whom I loved so much, in things that held no interest for him any more; things he no longer had the strength to fight, or rail against, or have an opinion about. It destroyed me.

I would leave the house I'd grown up in, and park just outside the driveway and sob. I would cry because it was so useless. *I* was so useless. I couldn't mend any of it. We used to talk about everything except what it felt like to die. And I truly thought we would. I thought he'd confide in me. We were that close. I thought, being his elder daughter – the one he could count on to be matter-of-fact and practical, and the one with whom he shared a love of books and writing – he would share his fears with me. I genuinely thought he'd impart the final bit of the puzzle. To me. Explain the riddle of life. I thought I was the one. Thought I was special. I was the one who could take it. I was like a boxer; ready to take the blows for everyone else, ready to absorb them and shield the rest of my family from what they couldn't handle. I could filter out the crap and hand them all the acceptable version; the one they could tolerate. The movie version. But it never happened.

I would lie, holding his hand, and I would look out of the window over the treetops and make the tiniest of tiny talk. He had no energy and no will left, and I lacked the courage to do anything but placate him; to try to smooth out that weird, unfamiliar passage that exists between living and leaving. I wish, wish, wish – more than anything in the world – I'd just had the balls and the gumption to sick up all I wanted to say. But I didn't. And I'm not proud of that.

The only thing I'm proud of is that when Daddy had no appetite left, and we all became obsessed with him eating nutritious food – forcing him to pointlessly down mouse-bites of poached cod and spinach – I asked him what he really, really fancied to eat. He thought for a while and then said he wanted a perfectly ripe, white peach.

I drove to Marks & Spencer in Camberley and bought

ten packets of 'buy now, save for later' peaches. I peeled them all. I tested them. Their fuzzy, furry skins discarded with wanton abandon. I tasted them. I spat them out. And eventually I found one. The perfect peach. Fragrant. Drippingly juicy. One that tasted of France and lazy holiday breakfasts and times past. Happier days. I fed it to my dad in little morsels, as though he were a baby. My baby. And it was the last thing he ever ate. From then on, it was swabs of water to moisten his parched lips. Nil by mouth. But the peach went down. He savoured it.

I'm forever grateful I was able to find that peach, because every time I eat one now that he's gone, it's a gentle reminder. I taste him in that peach. He is my lovely, delicious bite of sheer pleasure.

Now I must rediscover old pleasures and learn to live with the inevitable daily health niggles. I call them the DHNs. Ultimately, most niggles turn out to be just hypochondriacal nothings, but post-cancer, normal aches and pains insidiously turn into knotweed of the brain. It doesn't matter how much you hack it back, dig it out, torch it, poison it, or raze it, the knotweed of doubt succeeds in burrowing its rhizomes deep into the darkness of irrationality. It's going to take a while for me to regain trust in my body. To take it for granted again. It's been unfaithful towards me for so long, it's as though all my neurotransmitters are tangled up.

Just as getting a cancer diagnosis requires a period of

adjustment, so too does feeling well again. And I mourn. I can't pretend I don't. I grieve the loss of innocence, and the safety I felt within my skin. The reliability.

Back in 2020, I likened my illness to a car that had broken down. I thought I'd get it towed to the garage and pick it up when it was mended. It seemed like a good analogy at the time. My car has come back, but it's still battered and dented. It's survived the impact of the car crash, but there's a fair bit of housekeeping left to attend to: cobwebs to dust off, and areas to restore to their former glory. Well, 'glory' might be a tad ambitious. There's a lot of body maintenance to deal with.

After I've finished having chemo and all the scan results have come through, my oncologist rings me at home. I am in bed, nursing a savage migraine; the fallout of fasting for my tests the previous day.

It turns out I'm not going to have radiotherapy, after all. Instead, I'm having a two-year course of cutting-edge 'belt and braces' immunology treatment that seeks out and zaps any lingering, wandering cancer cells. The waifs and strays. The die-hard partygoers. It will annihilate them.

The port remains. I must go into hospital every two months and have this infusion over a period of three hours. No hair loss. Minimal, if any, side effects. It's like a pension plan for cancer. I'm back with the gang again.

I didn't even know this was on the cards: 'chemo-lite', I call it.

*

And then my heart goes crazy again. After four of these new treatments.

I'm back in my shop, sitting cross-legged on the floor, pricing new stock. Nothing strenuous. Tilly is there, and so is Diana. It's two weeks before Christmas 2021 and although not back working full time, I'm happily dipping in and out of shopkeeping duties. Not quite skidding across the floor with busyness like before – in the old, pre-cancer days – but taking it relatively easy and leaving the heavy work to the others. I am sick of feeling an outsider and am edging my way back to full normality. Masked, still, but getting increasingly adventurous. My whole family is going to be together this Christmas. Glory, glory hallelujah.

BOOM!

My heart's speeding up. I don't say anything, but I put down the toys I'm pricing and stay very still, hoping I've made a mistake.

Boom! Boom!

I can't ignore it. I need to take the pills my cardiologist has given me in case this happens. 'Just carry them with you,' he said. 'Take one immediately. If it keeps playing up, take another.'

They are at home, and I've written 'heart attack pills' in big red letters on the box. So I don't forget what they're for. But I don't have them with me.

'Tills, would you call Dad and ask him to go to the bedroom and whizz over the box of pills beside the bed marked "heart attack",' I say nonchalantly, trying not to overly alarm her.

Johnnie can't find them. By now my heart has gone into total free fall. Pounding like a woodpecker. I feel very odd.

Diana flags a taxi and Tilly takes me home. I get the pills. Take two and lie on the sofa.

'I think perhaps I need to go to hospital,' I say sadly, after about ten minutes. 'The pills aren't working.'

I ring the chemo ward to explain that I'm coming in. I tell them I've taken my heart rate and it's 210.

'No, you're not coming in,' says the doctor in charge. 'You are absolutely not to get into a car. Forbidden. Much too risky. You are calling an ambulance immediately and going to whichever hospital they take you to. Put the phone down and call now. We can liaise with wherever they take you.'

Johnnie is so unnerved he's shaking. He can't dial the numbers. His fingers aren't working properly. SOS. 999. I take over. I'm calm, even though I know my heart is breaking again.

The ambulance arrives and they allow Tilly in with me. This will be the very first time I'm not alone in hospital. They put the sirens on and radio ahead to St Thomas' Hospital to expect me. It's an emergency.

'I'll be fine,' I say to Tilly, watching her ashen little face. 'Promise you. I'm Teflon.'

The paramedics are doing an ECG and giving me oxygen as we speed along. I'm cold. They cover me in a tinfoil blanket, like they give to runners after a marathon. I feel like such a turkey.

I stay in hospital for four hours while the doctors work their magic and send their findings back to my team at the Cromwell.

My cardiologist calls the next day, having read the reports, and tells me it will keep happening. 'I know this feels awful, but all you need is a minor operation to prevent it recurring. It's called an ablation. I do about four a day. You don't even have to have an anaesthetic; it's a very, very simple procedure.'

I'm over simple procedures. 'How simple?' I snap.

'We just go in, up through your groin, and basically break the circuit. Day patient job. You can even watch on the screen while I'm doing it.'

'No,' I say. 'I can't do that. I'm not brave enough. Sorry. I just can't. Forgive me.' I'm back to my old routine of apologising for not being brave enough. Don't have the balls to watch a tiny tube being threaded, through my groin, into my heart. Sorry.

'Okay,' he says. 'You can be put under, if that's what you'd prefer. Call my secretary and I'll see if I can fit you in before Christmas.'

Fuck my life.

Three days before Christmas Eve, I go back to the Cromwell and wait to be wheeled down to theatre. But I'm not wheeled down this time. I walk. This time I'm strong.

I sit outside the operating theatre waiting. I'm in an open-backed gown and I'm jiggling with nerves. Everything is so different this time. I'm totally present, for starters. I'm no longer floating up to the ceiling. I'm in the here and now. I'm not trying to defuse my emotions; to detach myself from what's happening. And I suddenly realise I could easily just get up and go. Leave. I don't need to do this if I choose not to. I could run away. Chicken out. I seriously contemplate doing just that. But then I remember, I'm not a coward.

To borrow Julia Roberts' memorable line to Hugh Grant in *Notting Hill*, 'I'm just a girl, sitting outside an operating theatre, waiting to get my heart fixed.' I want my heart fixed. I don't want to be broken. I can do this.

Matt, my cardiologist, comes out to get me. In I go. Up on to the operating table, inflatable mattress heated beneath me, lights on, team introducing themselves, and paper knickers off.

'We just have to quickly shave half your pubic hair in order to insert the small wire up into your groin, and then we'll put you out,' he explains.

As though it's the most normal thing in the world to shave only half a bush. In front of four people.

I look up at the ceiling. I don't float. I look.

'You'll feel the tiny sting of a local, followed by a wee bit of tugging, and then we'll put you under completely.'

A few hours later and I'm half-bushed and home in time for tea.

Everything is tickety boo. With any luck, no more *booms*.

*

Having spent the last eighteen months looking backwards at my life, it's finally time to cast my sights forward
again.

Strangely, scientists have recently discovered there
may be a relationship between fond memories – such as
those triggered by a childhood classroom or a favourite
packet of sweets – and the areas of our brain that perceive
and register pain. Nostalgia and our autobiographical
memory can act as a painkiller.

I know this to be true. The past is where I sought refuge when I was sick. But now I must embrace the future.

I know it was science and love that saved me. Nothing
else. The love and support of my family and friends. The
brilliant doctors and nurses. The kindness of strangers
who reached out to me in the depths of the night. And
the meds.

You did it. All of you. You got me through.

It was love, actually.

Richard Curtis, thank you from the bottom of my
heart, I salute you.

'And . . . action,' as my old dad would say.

Richard, I'm ready for my close-up.

EPILOGUE

Life. The condition that distinguishes animals and plants from inorganic matter, including the capacity for growth, reproduction, functional activity and continual change preceding death. Whoa. I just looked that definition up. Heavy. Non-negotiable. But I guess most of life is light until it's under siege and you begin to question it. Or it was to me. Death was abstract; something obviously unavoidable, but for most of my youth and early adulthood it remained a mirage that exclusively belonged to old age; a destination I naively imagined I would reach in my own time and under my own terms.

When I was very young, I never paused to contemplate the noose of parental fear that seeks to strangle those that love you the most. I was just cavalier and cunning; irritated by the safety precautions my parents put in place to keep me safe and alive. Youth is full of broken promises. Little lies one makes in order to reassure the adults. Get them off your back. Set you free.

'I will never hitch-hike, trust me,' I reassured mine when I was at High School in America. I did.

'I won't smoke/take drugs/have more than one drink. I know the rules,' I'd say without even having the decency to cross my fingers behind my back. 'I'm not an idiot.' And out into the night I'd go. The insouciant callowness of youth worn like an indestructible cloak of self-belief. I never once doubted my mortality.

But guess what? I survived. I grew up, got married, had children of my own. And here's where Philip Larkin makes a surprise appearance in the maternity ward. Within a nano-second of giving birth for the first time I got the fog of parental fear. Like a whisper of responsibility, the visceral noose of omnipresent danger was now firmly tethered around my own neck.

Life. For the last eighteen months I've snatched it. I've plucked it away from doom and gloom and compartmentalised it. Today. Today is what counts. I've imagined myself like Hugh Grant in *Notting Hill*. That scene where he mourns losing Julia Roberts and wanders down Portobello Road and the seasons magically morph from winter to spring to summer to autumn. From the snuggle and silence of snow to the shirtsleeves of summer. I've walked that road; gradually casting my sights up from the pavement to looking straight ahead. I've got the T-shirt, got the puffer jacket, put my dark glasses on and raised my face like a sunflower towards the open skies. I thought my new life would be savoured slowly but it surprised me by still speeding on by. When I was locked down and isolated and being chemo-ed I imagined that when I got better, I'd spend my days slowly figuring out the theory of relativity or absorbing *A Brief History of Time*, but it was the minutia of normality that occupied and thrilled me. The fact I'd mastered how to make soda bread or grow crocuses in a pot outside my front door or made wonky-shaped cookies and a sticky mess with my grandsons: these were the little achievements I cherished and scrapbooked and added to my pension plan of treasured memories like sandbanks stacked against the rising waters.

I travelled. I went to visit my sister in Los Angeles and drank green celery juice every morning and walked out of air conditioning to sit outside, sip coffee and brown my legs. I looked out across the suburban landscape of Beverly Hills as the breeze fluttered the palm trees and the seductive hum of impending heat rose across the horizon.

I went to France with hair that was just starting to sprout like cress from cotton wool and wore a swimsuit that covered my port and all of it was as magical as I remembered and as I wanted it to be. I used to dream I'd return to Manderley when I was withered and broken and weak and I did. I made it. Nothing had changed. Only me.

But I came to realise I'd never truly addressed the fact I'd come through a cyclone of landscape-altering storms. I numbed myself in order to pretend I hadn't been felled and petrified. I made myself live in the lovely present but glossed over the past; initially failing to acknowledge the creases that still existed. Maybe pretending isn't the right word. I compartmentalised everything without allowing for an overlap. It's all good and dandy to live in the present – and I've become very adept at it – but deep down I didn't allow myself to think of a future. I hoped I had one, but the 'what ifs' were always putting the brakes on my natural optimism. I was in limbo. I looked healthy, I acted healthy, I had my restless energy back, but I got unreasonably angry whenever my family reassured me that I was better because I felt I was back to managing their expectations. And their expectations differed from mine. I knew cancer intimately. They didn't. I knew cancer was an assiduous, bullying creep. Having cancer is like being in an abusive relationship with disease. Like it or not, you are the unwilling victim in an extremely unhealthy relationship. But you can't just slam the door and walk away. Cancer gives you medicinal Stockholm syndrome. You must keep going back for scans and tests which makes one's future switch from being a promise to that of a potential threat. There is no choice but to keep going back for another possible thrashing.

And lo and behold I got beaten up. Again. Having been in remission and spent the last eighteen months having my course of immunotherapy infusions as a 'belts-and-braces' precaution, I went for my bi-annual PET scan. No big deal. Life was sweet.

I'd just returned from a week in Spain. Tilly and Felix had got officially married in a London registry office and we'd followed it with a glorious, non-traditional, crazy, *Mamma Mia*-like, three-day celebration-extravaganza surrounded by 130 friends and family at Trasierra, an idyllic secret paradise just an hour outside of Seville. It was a non-conformist's wedding dream. Unforgettably magical. A service conducted in the hotel's cobbled courtyard by

Fabian Frankel – an actor friend of Tilly's – and eight-year-old Huck who made the newlyweds promise 'to always love one another and make each other laugh'. Good maxim vows to live by. The guests were all got up like exotic butterflies; floaty summer dresses that fluttered in golden hour's comedown heat of the early evening; the watered-down light that softly kisses everyone before drenching them in beauty. Tilly was led towards Felix by Johnnie, her in a simple white dress clutching a bunch of daisies, and her dad in a pair of box-fresh Nike Air Max. At eighty-eight I don't expect he necessarily imagined he would live to have that moment and I'm not convinced two years ago I did either. The Le Bon sisters sang 'Something' by the Beatles and it WAS a Richard Curtis movie. I'm sorry to be corny, but it was. A real block-buster. From dinner in the olive grove with one long table that seemed to snake as far as the eye could see, to moving speeches and a show-stopping, unexpected, irreverent rap by Archie. He stood up and brilliantly channelled that scene in *Succession* where the character Kendall Roy stands up to honour his father and ends up giving a totally outrageous and inappropriate roast. Archie truly missed his vocation. He has an innate ability to read the room and own the stage. Or on this occasion, the olive grove. He rewrote the words, took the mic and had the guests standing up on their chairs, waving their white napkins and chanting 'T-I-L-L-Y. Tilly is getting m-aa-rr-ied to F-E-E-L-Y'. You had to be there to appreciate both the gall and the brilliance. There were mad first dances to 'I'm Still Standing', many tequila shots and a 3 a.m. resurrection from sleep by Huck, who heard 'Mamma Mia' being played on the dance floor, got dressed and came to find me, because he knew it was my favourite dance turn. Everyone present was loved-up and living in the moment.

So, I was hirsute and glowing in the aftermath of one of the happiest days of my life when I returned to hospital for a routine top-up of immunotherapy after my scan.

'Oh Sarah, Dr Plowman wants you to halt your treatment and wait here until he's seen you. He needs to talk to you and discuss your scan results.'

Hello darkness my old friend. Here we go again. We're back to rolling in the deep. Halting. Stopping. Ceasing. That. Must. Mean. It's back. The slight backache I'd brushed off during the wedding patently wasn't due to lugging heavy luggage on to trollies. I'm about to get beaten up.

'Okay,' I said. 'How long will he be?'

'Hopefully not too long, but it may take a while because lots of roads are closed due to Her Majesty dying.'

'Okay,' I replied. My voice sounded far away and tinny. And I sat in the chemo room, jiggling. My mind was somersaulting. Flip-flopping. Good cop, bad cop. It's nothing. It's terminal. It's back. I'm fine. I'm going to go down. Help me. Help me be strong. Again. Please don't make me hijack my family and hold them hostage to happiness. Not again. I've got this. I think. I hope. I pray. Deep breaths.

A nurse I'd never met before brought in a tin of Quality Street and a cup of tea and I helped myself to two fat purple-wrapped Brazil nuts.

'You need to talk me off the ledge,' I confided in him. 'I'm scared. What does "halting treatment" mean exactly?'

'Let me go and get your notes,' he said. 'I'm not familiar with them.'

He came back and held my hand. 'Listen,' he said. 'I've treated patients for twenty years with non-Hodgkin's lymphoma. It may keep coming back to bite you, but it's unlikely it will kill you.'

Okay. Okay. I get it. Breathe. Cancer. There may never be a definite line drawn in the sand. There might well be many sequels. And this is round two. A small patch has shown up in my diaphragm. More biopsies. More waiting for results. Delays in getting the results due to the Queen's funeral. The verdict: twenty sessions of radiotherapy. Once more unto the breach. Ten minutes a day lying on a cold steel mattress with a machine silently circling my waist. I chose to always ask if I could listen to Abba, played loudly. I'd dance my feet in time to the music. 'Waterloo'. 'S.O.S'. 'Take a Chance on Me'. 'Super Trouper'.

Today is New Year's Day. I have a six-week wait until my next scan. Six weeks to see if I've been successfully zapped. I'm still the impatient patient. When I first got ill, I sought refuge in my past. The past was safe. Yet if I've learnt anything over the last two years it's that although life can only really be understood backwards, it must be lived forwards at full throttle. Otherwise, there is no point to any of it. And I will. I will. I intend to keep to that resolution. Fuck you, cancer. Catch me if you can.

THE END

ACKNOWLEDGEMENTS

Without my family I couldn't have got through any of this. They were – and are – my oxygen.

J-Cat – the kindest, most loving husband that ever existed. He's always let me be me, and never more so than during this period of my life. I love him for so many reasons, but especially the fact he had to Sellotape a big A4 piece of paper to our kitchen counter saying NON-HODGKINS LYMPHOMA, to remind him what was wrong with me, after he told two friends I had a completely different cancer. Keeping it real.

My children and their husbands/partners. India and Sean, Archie and Nisha, Tilly and Felix. You all went above and beyond. Standing on my doorstep in the freezing cold, making me spinach and watercress soup every week, ordering the occasional Five Guys on Deliveroo, knowing I'd only be able to eat two mouthfuls, lending me their dog – Hank – to keep me company, and never once laughing at my wigs.

My mother, who had to isolate and lock-down alone aged eighty-seven, who got a car to drive her up to London in sheet rain and sat outside my house on the pavement just so she could physically see me. She rang me every single day and refused to accept the fact I might not get better. I love her for her eternal optimism.

My sister Emma, who made herself available in America 24/7. I could (and did) ring her late at night when I had 'the fear' when no one else was awake and she would talk to me for hours. She also spoilt me rotten and would send me a parcel every single week I was having treatment. Thanks to her I virtually have a new wardrobe and enough treatments for dry mouth and ulcers to last a lifetime. I missed her dreadfully and love her hugely.

Without my great friend Anya and Emma this book would have disappeared into the ether. I am a total Luddite and incapable of successfully saving anything I've written. They were both self-appointed keepers of the gate. Everything I wrote I sent to them in increments and Anya created a file and printed out my pages for me. She also rang me without fail every single day (and still does) and she is the most positive, practical woman in the world and I love her with all my heart.

My glorious grandsons Huck and Billy, who both make me want to live forever.

'Be kind' is a mantra I strive to live by. The following people were exceptionally kind to me. It's easy to be kind and thoughtful once or twice when someone is going through a crisis, but truly appreciated when they go the distance. Diana, Victoria, Rita, Nina, Felicity, Mark, Kathryn, Lily, Sam, Graham, Stevo, Charlotte, Celestia, Jo and Ben, Eric, Phoebe, Fiona, Susie Amy, Fiona, Suzy Murphy, Gina, Emma Ainley, Nick, Geordie, Nicola, Alexander (my glorious step-son), Keren and Fergie. Reidy (who lent me Gordon to drive me to hospital – such a generous and thoughtful lifesaver), my Book Club, Christopher and Sarah, every one of my followers on Instagram, especially those also with cancer, my amazing and stalwart American friends Barbara and Billy, Rita Milch, and of course Tricia Brock, who organised one of the most memorable and moving nights of my life. Louise for always making me laugh and keeping me grounded and endlessly surrounding me with beautiful flowers. Adrian and Mil, I will never stop missing you. You both taught me so much.

Elton and David for taking my mother under their wing and making her part of their Covid bubble. I would have lost my mind were it not for you two. You are both amazing examples of 'paying it forward'. Thank you. I am forever grateful.

My amazing agent Caroline Michel and the entire team at Headline who made the whole experience of publishing this book nothing but a joy. Sarah, Louise and Feyi – you are the best.

And lastly, I'd like to thank my oncologist, Nick Plowman, all my doctors, nurses and the entire chemo team. You gave me nothing but care, comfort and hope. I am forever in your debt.